PHYSICIAN, HEAL THYSELF

What Every Practitioner
Should Know About
Alternative Medicine

by Richard Sarnat, M.D.

PHYSICIAN, HEAL THYSELF
An Herbal Free Press Book VII- MCMVC

Cover Design by David Bordow, Golden Creative Group
Interior Text Design by Sally Nichols
Production by Mullein Graphics
Transcription, Initial Editing by Leslie J. Kenyon
Copyeditor Lida Stinchfield

Library of Congress Catalog Card Number 95-77514

ISBN Number 0-9639297-2-0

Printed in the United States of America.

Contents

Dedication

To everyone who has been,
and will be infirm.

Forgive those who do not know that
they do not know.

Acknowledgements

While any list of acknowledgements will, by its very nature, contain unfortunate omissions, I would like to express my appreciation to the following people nonetheless:

Norma Wagner, Ph.D. Asst. Dean of Admission Rush Medical College during the 1970s – Thank you for having the vision to accept older and more varied applicants as part of the student population.

Dr. Jeff Salloway Ph.D. – Thank you for broadening my medical education by presenting alternative medical therapies as part of the basic curriculum at Rush Medical College.

Dr. Andrew Pasminski Prof. of Chiropractic and Naprapathy – For being the perfect role model of an alternative medical physician.

Michael Kenyon, Sarah Kenyon, & Loree Popp – For being role models who demonstrate living proof of the power of alternative health care.

Paul Schulick , N.H. Med. – For his endless inspiration and creativity in the field of the health-food industry.

Gail Zimmerman & Carol Sarnat, my sisters – For the many years I tortured them at the family dinner table with endless philosophical discussion that brought them to the verge of tears.

Judith Eleanor Sarnat, my mother – For her unconditional love, for putting up with my father, and for passing along to me her love of gardening.

Leonard Arthur Sarnat, MD my father – For being an excellent role model as to all of the positive aspects of an allopathic physician.

Maharishi Mahesh Yogi – For providing a straightforward technique for the development of perfect health.

Special thanks to Seth I. Kaplan, M.D., Robert Kennedy, and to all the wonderful friends worldwide who have inspired and guided me through various phases of my personal spiritual growth.

Foreword

Like most physicians, I went into medicine with an altruistic drive to help others. I was propelled by the hopeful idea that through good science, combined with carefully chosen interventions, I could help others overcome "dis-ease". While my mind was wrestling with questions of my future medical practice, however, my body was wrestling health issues. Other than monthly migraines, my earlier healthy status had been without question, with the specter of illness being either a curious puzzle to be solved or viewed only in the context of what one does to help others. Stress, an awful diet, and what was then unknown bacteria had likely invaded my gut. A difficult period followed, one in which medically-accepted treatments were attempted but proved futile. While illness wreaked havoc with my body, I encountered the most powerful lesson of my clinical training. I had begun the search for gentle ways to turn on the immune system so that my body could heal itself. Before I could begin the task of reforming my own approach to medical care, I was forced to "re-form" me.

From that time to this, a period of some 20 years, I have been thrust into a personal search that has led me outside and beyond the walls of medical school. It began with my study of stress and behavioral medicine including biofeedback and cognitive restructuring, to Chinese medicine including acupuncture, to other traditional body-mind and physical therapies from the East, to botanical (herbal) medicine, and to an extensive investigation into nutrition's affect on disease, particularly its role in cancer prevention and treatment. This latter topic, though now timely, was considered quite radical in my early years of study. I also did something else that was relatively unheard of: instead of merely looking at ill-being, I spent several years observing and evaluating those who overcame illness as well as those who had been blessed with optimal health, searching for commonly-held factors that contributed to wellness.

Recovered and immersed in clinical practice, I gradually implemented the most useful of the innovative tools I had studied. I prudently developed a staff of caring professionals whose intellectual curiosity sustained and enlivened my own. We investigated ways to assess each patient's clinical needs and individually tailor a comprehensive treatment plan for those under our care. For example, conventional cancer treatments — radiation, chemotherapy, and surgery — cause nutritional and immunological deficits of great biological significance, owing to both protein-calorie malnutrition and specific vitamin and mineral deficiencies. While this fact has been widely recognized, responses to it have differed and, with little exception, worthwhile attempts to address it have mostly been ignored. Assisted by university colleagues, I began with a dietary regimen consisting of foods selected to improve the diet's potential for tumor inhibition. Among the aims of the dietary regimen are those of maximizing response to conventional modes of treatment, diminishing side effects, and promoting quantity and quality of life.

Of the three conventional treatments, radiation therapy appears to produce the longest lasting immune impairments. It often causes fatigue and anorexia and can actually impede nutrient depletion. Damage to immune cells after radiation includes excessive destruction of small lymphocytes and impaired responsiveness of peripheral blood lymphocytes to antigens. Chemotherapy is also quite harsh. The effects of chemotherapy on immune functions include suppression of the inflammatory response, suppression of antibody responses and proliferation of immune cells, as well as other deficits which last from a few days to several weeks. Chemotherapy not only causes alterations in taste, ulcerations of the gastrointestinal tract, and periods of nausea, vomiting, intestinal ileus or diarrhea, which can decrease food intake, but also may disturb renal and hepatic functions, leading to anorexia, protein synthesis depression and decreased serum albumin. Surgery, too, has broad consequences. Not only does it alter anatomy and physiology, it impairs gastrointestinal functioning, requires increased stress on nutrient stores, and commonly causes immunological suppression, a complication which can persist a month or more postoperatively. For the patient struggling with cancer, the combined nutritional and immunological impact of both the disease and its treatments are thus profound.

As I have noticed, although scientific research has shown that cancer treatments and the disease itself can impose severe nutritional stress on the body, and that all attempts should be made in order to avoid allowing the possibility of patients becoming malnourished during the treatment or else their treatment may become compromised, most conventional practices in the United States do not include vigorous programs of nutritional support which incorporate the most recent research results. On the other hand, while alternative dietary treatments for cancer contain potentially interesting elements which might be of preventive or therapeutic use, most of them indiscriminately advise against the use of conventional cancer treatments (such as chemotherapy, surgery, or radiation). Because these two approaches to care are in opposition to each other, the cancer patient is thrown into the "either/or" confusion of the war against cancer. Needlessly, I might add.

A more reasonable approach would be to insure that patients be clinically repleted — maintained on a nutrient rich, carefully monitored regimen — while undergoing traditional therapies. Such an approach would provide more than adequate intake of vitamins, minerals, fats, complex carbohydrates, and protein, such as might be provided in the alternative diets, but still have the full advantages of conventional cancer care. This approach would benefit patients since they would suffer less from subtle or obvious malnutrition induced by conventional tools. Thus, this approach, which is more than either conventional medicine or alternative medicine, is the direction my own medical practice has taken.

Although we are now well accepted within the academic environments where I teach and practice, there was, in the earlier years, profound skepticism among many of my colleagues regarding the clinical significance and lasting value of our work. There were two important issues that distinguished us from the usual disdain encountered by alternative centers. The first was that we rigorously *combined* the two worlds of conventional and alternative practice, selecting only the best of each. We grounded ourselves in the sound science of conventional medicine and then we developed reasonable and rational therapies that, due to their health-enhancing intentions, we termed "complementary care," a more accurate and less needlessly provocative designation than "alternative medicine". Happily, this combination of conventional and adjunctive therapies has withstood the test of time and has become our trademark. Secondly, we continued to pursue rigorous and scientific research in a results-oriented academic setting, research focused on corroborating our theories and substantiating our clinical work. It is these two factors which not only identify our own work, but are at the core of Dr. Sarnat's work in presenting educational substance for health practitioners in the field of alternative medicine.

As Richard has so aptly conveyed, it is no longer possible to avoid the fact that pluralistic approaches to medical care are here to stay. Just as lumpectomy, radiation therapy, and hydrazine sulfate have historically moved from the alternative to mainstream arena, so will others. It is both our responsibility and our calling as caregivers to chase down and investigate promising new and innovative treatments with an open mind. Dr. Sarnat's book is an excellent starting point for the practitioner beginning such an exploration.

But what is it that makes such an exploration worth considering? Isn't it that medicine has been forging ahead against the awful backdrop of the dismal failure of Nixon's 1971 "War on Cancer"? More troubling even that the lack of cures that came out of the billions of dollars spent, has been the shift toward a medical culture of "curegivers" focused mostly on looking for a magic bullet to destroy disease, instead of "caregivers" intent on preventing disease and assuring longer and better quality lives. Did we need to pursue one at the expense of the other? Surely it was not necessary that medical care become an either/or proposition.

If, in the end, the solutions we seek are to achieve results, then placing more of our attention and resources on "caregiving" may facilitate this. In fact, by utilizing tools of caregiving, we may gain the additional edge needed to overcome some of the most intractable ailments. Along the way we may, find some less invasive approaches for re-establishing health when health has been compromised, approaches that are not as awesome as a magic bullet but simpler, kinder, less costly, and provide comparable results as well. Isn't this what we agreed to pursue when we pledged to "do no harm"? After all, it was Hippocrates, himself, who instructed, "What you should put first in all the practice of our art is how to make the patient well; and if he can be made well in many ways, one should choose the least troublesome."

With the rapidly changing nature of medicine these days, a "re-formation" of medical practice must include more than merely the content and style of practice. Rather, an authentic "re-formation" must include the very thought and philosophy of healthcare, one that focuses at least as much on acquiring good health as it does on the treatment of illness. Such a change will alter the way we caregivers are viewed by the public. More importantly, it will also replenish us while restoring the very ideals that drew us to the profession in the first place.

It is with this vision in his heart and mind that Dr. Richard Sarnat has explored healthcare in this important and timely book. More precise with words than I, W.B. Yeats unwittingly summed up American healthcare and the intent of this book when he observed, "The voyage of discovery lies not in seeking new vistas but in having new eyes." May *your* new eyes find a new vision herein.

Keith I. Block, M.D.

Medical Director, Cancer Treatment Program,
and Chief, Nutritional & Behavioral Oncology,
 Edgewater Medical Center, Chicago
Director, Nutritional and Psychosocial Oncology,
 Midwest Regional Medical Center, Zion
Vice President of Chicago-Uptown Chapter,
 American Cancer Society
Medical Consultant on Nutritional-Oncology Research for the
 Office of Technology Assessment for the Congress of the
 United States
Research Assistant Professor, Medical Dietetics and Nutrition,
 University of Illinois
Clinical Instructor, University of Illinois College of
 Medicine, Chicago

January 27, 1995

Introduction

Physician, Heal Thyself is about the changes that we, as physicians, must make to adjust to a 21st-century health-care system.

It is becoming increasingly obvious that striving to be healthy in a system designed only to be disease free is not working. The growing signs of a consumer shift from orthodox medical care to the alternative health-care system are seen on a daily basis within the news media. My challenge to the current medical establishment is that we must alter our present product (allopathic medicine as it currently exists). Otherwise, I feel we will have an ever-eroding market share of potential patients. In other words, as in all competitive markets, it is time to decide whether we must truly "beat them or join them."

Historically, organized medicine under the direction of the AMA has adopted the tactic of "divide and conquer." However, with the historic court judgment in favor of chiropractic against the AMA, I believe it is obvious that this tactic is no longer useful.

It has never made sense to me that the wide diversity of health-care practitioners have failed to share their knowledge. I am suggesting it is no longer efficient to have various health-care systems in competition with one another. Rather, it is time to learn from each other and provide a unified product, which will be the best possible, available to the consumer. This will require that we take the best that each system has to

offer, discarding the mysticism and nonscientifically-verifiable compo-
nents that remain.

Most of all, it demands that we re-empower the patient as the
primary healer in contrast to ourselves, the physicians, or our other-
directed health-care system. It is my hope that by reading this book,
the health-care provider will understand the need to re-examine our
relationship to ourselves, our patients, our Natural World, and perhaps even our God knowing, ultimately, we are not gods.

1

Not Just Business As Usual

A Primer of "Alternative Medicine"

It is my intention in writing this book to document both a historical phenomenon, namely, the current revolution and crisis in health care delivery; and to provide a unique model or framework from which to understand the various forces that currently shape the health-care marketplace.

As a young student in my undergraduate career, I majored in philosophy. This was a most unusual major for a prospective doctor. Nonetheless, I feel it gave me a unique perspective for understanding the complexity of the world around me. Perhaps my greatest lesson as a philosophy student was to understand the importance of asking the right question.

Very often there is no right answer that can be agreed upon by a collection of experts. But if one does not know how to even pose the right question, then it is very clear that he does not understand the subject at hand. The question that lies before us is the following: What exactly is at the cause of the revolution in health care, and what is the basis of the current crisis?

To any objective observer it is obvious that something truly revolutionary is taking place in the consumer marketplace. By the government's own accounts, 35% of all patients are now utilizing "alternative health-care modalities," and approximately 75% of those doing so fail to inform their traditional physicians. In 1990 alone the *New England Journal of Medicine* estimates that over $14 billion was spent by consumers involved in alternative medicine.[1] This is an entirely consumer-driven revolution, spurred by dissatisfaction with traditional medical practices and their results.

Perhaps there is no more convincing evidence that this emerging movement has come of age than its having made the cover of *Time* magazine. What could be more indicative of mainstream America? The cover story of the November 4, 1991, edition was titled "The New Age of Alternative Medicine." Since these ground-breaking articles, even more significant changes have occurred in the power structure of medicine. In 1992 under the direction of Joe Jacobs, a physician who had been trained as a pediatrician, the National Institute of Health (NIH) began operating the Office of Alternative Medicine. The Office of Alternative Medicine has only a $2 million annual budget — roughly 1/50 of one percent of the total NIH budget — but it provides an unprecedented opportunity for practitioners of alternative medicine to try to demonstrate that their practices are scientifically valid.

In 1994 the National Institutes of Health announced it would fund research in the following areas:

- The use of acupuncture to treat depression
- Biofeedback as a treatment for pain control and diabetes
- Ayurvedic medicine (the traditional medicine of India) to treat Parkinson's disease
- The benefits of hypnosis in healing broken bones
- Music therapy for people with brain injuries
- Massage therapy for patients with the AIDS virus, postsurgical patients, and people with bone-marrow transplants
- Yoga for heroin addiction and obsessive compulsive disorder
- The effects of prayer on health

Unfortunately, like all entrenched bureaucracies, the current medical establishment is very slow to admit that there is a crisis in consumer faith, trust and acceptance of our established health-care system. Nor does it have any notion of how to solve it. For to truly get to the basis of current consumer dissatisfaction, an entirely new paradigm of medical-care needs to be understood, which is totally foreign to orthodox medical education as we know it today.

It is this new paradigm or model that will encompass both consumers' demands and expectations, as well as the larger reality of proper medical care, that I hope to contribute to in writing this book.

WHO IS THE CONSUMER?

I would assert that the main impetus for the revolution in health care is the fact that the consumer has undergone an evolutionary change. This should not be a surprising phenomenon, as the consumer is a natural part of the evolution of a society. There can be no doubt, despite many historians' attempts to trivialize it, that since the 1960s an enormous revolution has taken place in this country as well as the rest of the world.

One need only look at the growth of the natural-foods industry (health-food industry), the overwhelming popularity of health clubs, the heightened awareness of the dangers of tobacco usage, the growing awareness of contaminants and pollutants not only as a worldwide phenomenon, but as they affect our daily life and our personal health.

All of this has arisen within a milieu of even more profound political and socioeconomic changes, such as the cessation of the Cold War, the fall of the Soviet Union as an empire, the dissolution of the Berlin Wall, the new historical movement for peace in the Mideast, etc.

Public opinion polls, long circulated by the AMA in an attempt to inform its constituents, have revealed that consumer confidence and respect for their physicians have been eroding. It comes as no surprise to any practicing physician, such as myself, that we are no longer held in the esteem that physicians were one generation before us. Isn't this truly a paradoxical phenomenon, considering that the efficacy of our treatments has improved so greatly? Wouldn't common sense tell us that exactly the opposite should be so?

WHAT ARE WE AS PHYSICIANS DOING WRONG?

Never before in the history of mankind have physicians been able to neuroimage the brain with CAT scans and MRIs, to perform the wonders of microsurgery, and to dissect the etiology of genetically based diseases, as well as a host of other miraculous procedures that reduce the suffering of mankind in ways heretofore unimagined. Yet the fact remains that the market, driven by consumer demand and perception, is going in the opposite direction. What can account for this?

In the late 1970s, when I was a medical student, a new word appeared in my medical education. That word, or concept, was *holistic*. The term *holistic* (meaning wholeness of body and mind) derives from the theory of holism, which says that a living organism has a reality other than the sum of its constituent parts.

It became clear to both the medical students and professors at that time that a certain dissatisfaction was growing among a small patient population. We suddenly had a population of patients who were not content to treat isolated disease phenomena as they appeared. Compared to the average patient population, these consumers were much more aware of the inability of current allopathic medicine to provide a unified perspective in the treatment or solution of their problems.

As medical technology progressed and overspecialization became the norm, the tendency to fragment medical care into easily definable and quantifiable entities further exacerbated this problem. Dissatisfied with the inability to receive treatment that they considered holistic, this segment of the patient population looked elsewhere. They sought out nontraditional sources of medical care such as chiropractic, herbal medicine, homeopathy, and acupuncture to provide them with techniques to become healthy.

For this patient population it was no longer satisfactory to treat each disease symptom in isolation. These patients intuitively realized, perhaps long before their medical practitioners, that a piecemeal treatment of disease symptoms without a unifying theory connecting the entire body was not satisfactory.

Even more revolutionary, this patient population truly aspired to *be healthy*. Former patient populations had only striven to be disease free. The idea of aspiring toward and achieving a true state of health is a concept wholly new to traditional allopathic medicine.

More startling is the fact that we, as allopathic physicians, have not conceptualized or defined what a healthy person should be. Rather, it is our specialty to attack the specific manifestation of a disease (e.g., a cardiac arrest) and successfully bring the patient through the disease episode. Only recently have we developed cardiac rehab programs that aim at changing the total person in order to avoid a recurrence of the problem based on the patient's lifestyle.

Thus, the consumer had evolved to a higher expectation of health care than our system was able to deliver. And while leading psychologists, such as Abraham Maslow,[2] provided a basis for this type of conceptualized thinking (as evidenced by his work on "self-actualized individuals"), physiologically based medical curriculum had no such concept or methodology.

Nor are these problems unique to the United States. They exist to some extent in almost every country of the world. They undergo different forms in each country, based on economics, social customs, geography, national pride, scientific attitudes, legal differences, and even politics. Clearly, the world as a whole has failed to organize the sum total of its health-care experience into a unified body of knowledge that provides easy access, high effectiveness, and a low percentage of side effects.

What Changes Must We as Physicians Make?

Recently the director general of the World Health Organization (WHO), after a worldwide study by two international health agencies, declared that if the health needs of the world are to be adequately met by the year 2000, orthodox Western medicine will not be able to achieve the goal. It was the opinion of WHO that the traditional medical systems of all countries should be utilized, retaining the very best elements of each and removing the ineffective ones. In other words, if the world's populace is to achieve a state of "health" in the near future, alternative health-care systems rather than orthodox Western medical systems will be leading the way.[3]

This last paragraph should come as a shock to most physicians and patients alike in the United States today. To be perfectly honest, I, too, was unaware of the recommendations of WHO until I undertook preparations for this book.

The next question is obvious. On what basis did WHO reject ortho-dox Western medicine in favor of the more traditional medical systems of ancient civilizations? I believe the answer has many levels, and each level will lead us closer to the truth of the cause of our current crisis in health-care delivery.

Obviously, the first level most easily seen is that of economics. West-ern medical therapy is based on pharmaceutical intervention, which is an extremely expensive option. Very few countries can afford the cost of modern pharmaceutical development and modern technological advances. In fact, I believe it has become increasingly clear that our country itself cannot afford it. At present, one seventh of all hospital days in the United States are devoted to the care of drug toxicity, at a yearly cost of $3 billion, as reported by a U.S. government task force on prescription drugs in 1969.[4]

Nor do we still believe that a completely selective drug, or "magic bullet," which can home in on its target, while leaving intact the sur-rounding physical environment, is possible. Absolute selectivity in a drug is never absolute. In fact, since 1960 adverse drug reactions of all different kinds have become so common that a new disease etiology, called "iatrogenic" or doctor induced, has come into recognition. The use of this term is so commonplace today that we forget that it was first proposed by Ivan Illich in 1975. Illich, a brilliant and provocative social commentator, opened his attack on allopathy in his book *Medical Nemesis* with the statement: "The medical establishment has become a major threat to health."[5]

Unfortunately, this disturbing statement is all the more alarming when one scrutinizes the ethical performance of the pharmaceutical industry. It would be nice to believe that all companies marketing and making fortunes out of drugs are well aware of their heavy responsibili-ties to the public. However, much evidence suggests that they are more aware of their responsibilities to their shareholders, and their marketing techniques are those designed to produce a profit at almost any cost.

In 1976, in his book *The Drugging of the Americas*, author Milton Silverman showed that "multinational drug companies say one thing about their products to physicians in the United States, and another thing to physicians in Latin America."[6] A perfect example is the fact that in countries where no FDA exists to police them, well-known

U.S. companies have been found to dump their more dangerous pharmaceuticals.

In 1970, for instance, Parke Davis was marketing Chloromycetin to Mexico and central Latin American countries for a wide range of uses: dysentery, tonsillitis, ear infections, phlebitis, ulcerative colitis and syphilis. While at the same time, under the police scrutiny of the FDA, this drug was to be used only for life-threatening infections within the United States.

Chloromycetin is a drug that is effective in a certain type of meningitis caused by the H. influenza bacillus, as well as in diseases caused by typhoid and similar germs. In such situations, Chloromycetin is often the only antibiotic that will work. But Chloromycetin also has the not uncommon fatal side effect of interfering with the bone marrow's production of blood cells.

When a person's life is at stake anyway, this is an acceptable risk to take. But if a child is suffering from a minor infection, risking the depression of the child's bone marrow is certainly not warranted. Nonetheless, this was the drug unleashed upon unsuspecting markets outside of the United States.

However, the economics of the pharmaceutical industry is only one level that has gone awry in our Western medical orientation. The deeper and more fundamental level is that Western science has attempted to cure man by controlling nature.

In his book *Medical Nemesis*, Ivan Illich describes this attempt of man to control nature by the usage of the Greek term *nemesis:*

> "I will designate the self-reinforcing loop of negative institutional feedback by its classical Greek equivalent and call it *medical nemesis.* The Greeks saw gods in the forces of nature. For them, nemesis represented divine vengeance visited upon mortals who infringe on those prerogatives the gods enviously guard for themselves. Nemesis was the inevitable punishment for attempts to be a hero rather than a human being. Like most abstract Greek nouns, Nemesis took the shape of a divinity. She represented nature's response to *hubris:* to the individual's presumption in seeking to acquire the attributes of a god. Our contemporary hygienic hubris has led to the new syndrome of medical nemesis. I believe

that the *reversal of nemesis* can come only from within man and not from yet another managed (heteronomous) source depending once again on presumptuous expertise and subsequent mystification."[7]

We have attempted to *control* nature by the use of therapeutic intervention. How different this outlook is from the other philosophies of traditional medicine (East Indian/Chinese) that propose to cure man by harnessing nature's power, not by controlling it.

We will find that all of the alternative medical systems that will be reviewed later in this book have a common denominator in that they treat causes rather than symptoms. This is because they treat people as whole entities — and not just their diseases. The most important concept that the alternative medical systems share in common is that the human body has an incredible capacity to heal and rejuvenate itself if given the opportunity and proper circumstances to do so.

The various alternative medical systems provide different situations that promote the body's self-healing, as opposed to pharmaceutical intervention, which controls symptom manifestations. This is a subtle but all-important philosophical difference. As we will discover in the subsequent chapter on ancient medical traditions, the basis of Ayurveda (traditional East Indian medicine) is the belief that disease is cured by unlocking the latent intelligence within our physiology.

Like arrested adolescents, we in orthodox Western medicine are out to conquer disease and the world on our own terms. Deluded by the apparent power of modern technology and scientific advancement, we erroneously believe that we can control and bend all of nature to our whim. The world environmental movement has learned that this is clearly not the case. In fact, the more industrialized and sophisticated we become (e.g., the nuclear industry), the more dangerous and risky the side effects to the planet.

How similar is our increasing wariness of nuclear energy and our new romance with renewable energy sources? The current attempt to develop renewable energy sources is motivated by the exact same belief structure that now motivates the world to change its medical orientation: Nuclear energy, like Western medicine, is not safe. It is clearly not safe for the planet, as Three Mile Island and Chernobyl remind us, and it is clearly not safe for the patient, as government statistics regarding drug side effects bear out. More traditional forms of energy are being sought out on a daily basis, which attempt to harness the world's power in a nondangerous fashion.

Likewise, the future of medicine, according to WHO, will be to harness these various alternative medical systems that propose to cure not by controlling nature, but by coexisting with our own nature in a more harmonious fashion.

Only from divorcing ourselves from the natural world around us could such a horrible situation arise as we find ourselves in today. We, as human beings, are part of the natural world. Ivan Illich correctly points out that man is the only animal whose evolution has been conditioned by adaptation on more than one front. Once mankind successfully overcame predators and the forces of nature, he then had to cope with the use and abuse of power by others of his own kind.

Animals adapt through evolution in response to changes in their natural environment. Only in man does challenge become conscious and this adaptive process become a volitional pursuit. Mankind is the sole being who can and must redesign himself to limits when he becomes aware of them. A conscious response to painful sensations, to impairment, and to eventual death is part of man's coping ability.[8]

It is my contention that mankind has recently exceeded these limits in its attempt to control health with almost a godlike zeal. Until the present time, medicine attempted to enhance what occurs in nature. It fostered the tendency of wounds to heal, of blood to clot, and of bacteria to be overcome by natural immunity. Now medicine tries to engineer the dreams of reason.[9] The question is whether this reason has transgressed the limits imposed upon us by nature, whether in our "hubris" we have violated deeper laws of nature. (I know of no analogy to illustrate this better than the predicament we now find ourselves in with regard to nuclear energy.)

Once again, I believe it is time for man to correctly adapt to the powers he has unleashed, both on the health-care front and in the field of physics. It is time for us to rediscover our place within the natural world and, by doing so, learn to contact nature's healing forces from within us.

There are now many professional organizations such as the American College of Advancement in Medicine, the American Association of

Acupuncture, and the American Association of Orthomolecular Medicine that represent Western allopathic physicians and other practitioners who are beginning to incorporate specific alternative therapies into their more orthodox practices.

While the existence of these professional organizations is exciting, their constituency represents a very small percentage of the total number of practicing allopathic physicians in our country today. It is difficult to believe that we as physicians have become so short-sighted historically as to ignore our own basic nature in the healing process. Nonetheless, that is the position in which we now find ourselves.

Only a narrow view of reality based on limited awareness can account for such poor judgment. According to Jean Piaget, the father of developmental psychology, children expand their powers of abstract conceptualization as their central nervous systems evolve. This is an age-specific development allowing concepts, such as life, death, physical causation, and conservation of matter, to evolve. To quote Piaget, "The child is a being whose principal activity is adaptation and who is seeking to adapt itself not only to the adult who surrounds it but to nature itself."[10] Our ability to adapt to nature is what we mean by the term *intelligence.*

Another way of looking at this is summarized by the ancient philosophical dictum: Knowledge is structured in consciousness. As one's physiology (central nervous system) develops, one's consciousness or awareness develops. Increasing knowledge creates greater organizing power and enhances successful decision making. Like the young child who adapts to his new environment through the evolution of his abstract intelligence, I now believe that mankind as a whole is adapting to the new realities of the technological age.

The current revolution in health care is nothing more than the evolution of medicine. It is humanity's attempt to adapt properly to the natural world in which we find ourselves. Medicine's future course is no more than a shift in orientation from within our own potentialities.

The philosophies of healing we will discover as we review the various chapters of this book are nothing new. Rather, they are observations that have been empirically tested throughout the ages by various traditional medical systems.

> *A famous Chinese proverb says, "To find new
> things, first look for the old things.*

In the next few chapters, we will briefly review the alternatives available to the health-care consumer seeking alternative medical care. Entry points into the alternative health-care system include chiropractic, naprapathy, homeopathy, ancient Chinese and Indian medicines, and naturopathy to name a few.

I will try my best in the following chapters to provide an overview of each of these medical systems. Certain sections may receive more emphasis, depending on previous experience with a particular system and the evaluation of its relative importance to the whole. I hope the reader will forgive this obvious bias, which certainly exists despite the author's endeavor for objective scientific neutrality.

It is not my intention to debate the validity of one modality of treatment or philosophy of treatment over another. Nor is it my intention to validate the legitimacy of any particular treatment at all. Rather, I believe it is very important to familiarize the new medical practitioner with the current world of alternative choices and the consumer's rationale for making these choices.

It is my hope that the readers, especially current health-care providers, will review this information with an open mind and suspend judgment until the book's conclusion. Perhaps it will be helpful to remind ourselves just how much orthodox Western medicine is an art and not a science.

We need look no further than to orthodox Western-trained physicians, such as Dr. Robert Mendelsohn, who in his book *Confessions of a Medical Heretic* has reminded us of the illusion of our current medical certainties:

> "I no longer believe in modern medicine. . . . I believe that modern medicine's treatments for disease are seldom effective, and that they're often more dangerous than the diseases they're designed to treat.
>
> "I believe the dangers are compounded by the widespread use of dangerous procedures for nondiseases.
>
> "I believe that more than ninety percent of modern medicine could disappear from the face of the earth — doctors, hospitals, drugs, and equipment — and the effect on our health would be immediate and beneficial.
>
> "I believe that modern medicine has gone too far, by

using in everyday situations extreme treatments designed for critical conditions. . . . modern medicine can't survive without our faith, because modern medicine is neither an art nor a science. It's a religion."[11]

Although I quote Dr. Mendelsohn to jar the reader into the type of intellectual honesty necessary to pursue this book, I do not share his complete condemnation of orthodox Western medicine as a whole.

Dr. Mendelsohn's book carries the tone of a physician who is angry and betrayed by a philosophical system in which he once had complete faith. While I sympathize with his outrage and disappointment at modern medicine's track record, to discard all of medicine's scientific advancements is ludicrous. Rather, as he alluded to, critical treatments must be reserved for critical situations.

The apparent failure of modern medicine is not its inability to be successful in curing all disease, but rather its fundamental dishonesty in believing it can do so. Failing to admit its own inherent limitations, it has not availed itself of the wealth of information offered by the various alternative medical systems.

It is time we realize that critical intervention should be limited to critical care issues only. As this comprises approximately ten percent only of all health care, we are left with a void that must be addressed anew.

The alternative health-care system is well equipped as a starting place to look for answers in the arena of nonemergency care and ultimately the pursuit of good health. But in order to listen, we must open our minds to the available data that centuries of empiric documentation afford. This knowledge of how to heal the human body and mind, acquired over the millennia, cannot be discounted merely because we are now living in a technologically oriented society. We, the providers of orthodox Western medicine, must stop our slander of quackery while hiding behind the veil of modern scientific research.

With this task in mind, the book will conclude with my personal attempt to synthesize a new philosophy for understanding the relationship that each of these disciplines has to our current knowledge and to the health-care delivery system as a whole. It is a model/philosophy that has allowed me to understand my role both as a consumer and as a practitioner over the past fifteen years.

2

Health-Food Industry/Naturalistic Health Movement

The fact that the health-food industry has evolved into a multibillion dollar business over the past thirty years is perhaps the greatest testament to the revolution in health care currently taking place. And while most health-food consumers naively assume that this originated from the "back to nature" movement of the 1960s, nothing could be further from the truth. The concept of a naturalistic health-care philosophy can be historically traced back in the modern era to Adolph Just (1838-1936), who authored the book *Return to Nature*. He is considered one of the pioneers of naturopathy, a medical system reviewed in detail in the next chapter.

Gaylord Hauser, who popularized yoghurt and wheat germ in the United States in the 1930s, was also a central figure in the development of the health-food industry. But the health-food movement is much broader than the array of products we have come to associate with it. Health-food stores became popular nationwide because they filled a void for naturalistic healing that the orthodox medical establishment failed to address. In a very real sense, these small, often quaint apothecaries provide a physical location that the local alternative health-care community can identify as a sanctuary of shared ideals. If this last postulation strikes the reader as having political undertones, it is meant to.

Ivan Illich promotes the hypothesis that recovery from societywide iatrogenic disease is a political task, not a professional one. He believes it must be based on a grass-roots consensus regarding the balance between the civil liberty to heal and the civil right to equitable health care. It is his contention that during the last generations, the medical monopoly encompassing health care has expanded without checks and has encroached on our liberty with regard to our own bodies.

"Health" is, after all, an everyday word that is used to designate the intensity with which individuals cope with their internal states and their environmental conditions. What could be more intimate to oneself than to be in tune with one's own health status? According to Illich, the failure of our present medical system is its promotion of other-directed health care (hospital based and doctor controlled) rather than a system that promotes individual education and autonomous healing:

> "In part at least, the health of a population depends on the way in which political actions condition the milieu and create those circumstances that favor self reliance, autonomy, and dignity for all, particularly the weaker. In consequence, health levels will be at their optimum when the environment brings out autonomous personal, responsible coping ability. Health levels can only decline when survival comes to depend beyond a certain point on the heteronomous (other-directed) regulation of the organism's homeostasis. Beyond a critical level of intensity, institutional health care — no matter if it takes the form of cure, prevention, or environmental engineering — is equivalent to systematic health denial."[1]

If Illich's hypothesis is true, the job of future physicians and the health-care system is to *re-empower the patient*. This calls for less reliance upon physician-directed activities and greater reliance upon individual autonomous healing.

For Illich, this transformation is not just a question of health-care philosophies. It is a political issue that rocks the very foundation of our social structure. He feels "the medical and paramedical monopoly over hygienic methodology and technology is a glaring example of the political misuse of scientific achievement to strengthen industrial rather than personal growth."[2] He further highlights the danger of this phenomenon by describing it as a radical monopoly.

> A radical monopoly goes deeper than that of any one corporation or any one government . . . when hospitals draft all those who are in critical condition, they impose on a society a new form of dying. Ordinary monopolies corner the market; radical monopolies disable people from doing or making things on their own.[3]

Make no mistake about it, the health-food industry is a political movement. It forms the rallying point around which the clients of alternative medicine hope to regain control of their own health care. While your basic, everyday consumer found in the average health-food store may not verbalize his feelings with the eloquence and venom of Illich, alternative health-care consumers do share his ideals. Health-food stores are a source of educational materials as well as consumer products. Many provide bulletin boards full of advertisements for alternative health-care practitioners and act as ad hoc bookstores for alternative health-care publications. In short, they fulfill a social and political function for the reestablishment of individual autonomous healing over the form of bureaucratic institutionalized healing exemplified by mainstream medicine today.

Let us begin in this chapter to review the basic philosophical beliefs that underlie the alternative health-care systems. We will continue in subsequent chapters to show even more formal, systemized bodies of knowledge that all propose to re-empower the patient as the primary health-care agent in contrast to our present physician-directed system.

One of the main tenets of naturalistic healing philosophy is the concept of digestive autotoxicity. According to this belief, an unhealthy diet is at the root of most disease states. This improper diet leads to an imbalance in the nervous system created by the impurities or toxins of the digestive system, which autointoxicate the body. The source of this autointoxication is an inefficiency of the digestive system. A sluggish digestive system with a longer transit time increases the amount of time that an individual toxin is exposed to the body. Conversely, an efficient and rapid digestive system with a quick transit time will effectively eliminate toxic waste products from the body without allowing them time to autointoxicate it.

I remember, as a young intern, attending a lecture on medical epidemiology by Dr. Burkitt (the physician who is credited with discovering Burkitt's lymphoma). Dr. Burkitt at this time was an elderly physician who had retired from clinical practice in order to disseminate startling epidemiological facts he had discovered while practicing medicine in Africa. Dr. Burkitt noticed during his tenure in Africa that all of the common industrialized Western diseases such as appendicitis, diverticulitis, systemic hypertension, diabetes mellitus, and colon cancer were virtually unknown in the wilds of Africa. It was his conviction that the variable responsible for these widespread differences in disease patterns was the factor of diet.

As we have more recently discovered, a low fiber/high meat diet makes the process of digestive autotoxicity more common. This basic scientific discovery is now readily known to the lay person as large food companies have begun advertising high-fiber/low-fat products.

Parenthetically, it is interesting to note that while the concept of digestive autotoxicity is not the main foundation of either East Indian or Chinese medicine, it is certainly a core belief to both.

For the naturalistic practitioner, however, this is the foundation of his medical philosophy: Thus, most regimens directed at preserving the health of the patient incorporate high-fiber diets, the use of herbal colonic stimulants or age-old remedies such as castor oil or olive oil. These lubricate the digestive tract and promote quicker transit time.

A common remedy prescribed in today's market is the use of flax seeds, which are soaked and drunk for their additional bulk and promotion of digestion. Another tenet of this belief system includes the belief that organic fruits and vegetables are healthier than commercially produced foodstuffs, as they have less risk of contaminants to the body itself.

For the same reason, true naturalists will tend to be vegetarians, believing that the anatomical configuration of the digestive tract and lack of large canine teeth illustrate that man is meant to be a vegetarian and not a carnivore. Their understanding is that the addition of meat to the diet only promotes increased toxins in the system since meat is, after all, decaying flesh.

This is further aggravated in the more industrial era by the hordes of chemicals and fertilizers passed on to us through the food chain as well as the overall stressful conditions to the animal, which take place during its forced life span and the manner of slaughter.

The naturalistic physician and client will try to avoid all allopathic drugs whenever possible, as they believe these treatments, such as the use of commercial pharmaceuticals, are very strong and may have significant potential side effects. Unfortunately, for all of the modern medical miracles that pharmaceuticals can achieve, their inadvertent side effects are a very real issue. It warrants mentioning again that one seventh of all hospital days are devoted to the care of drug toxicity, at a yearly cost of $3 billion.

The fear of the naturalist is that any time the natural harmony of the system is disrupted through the use of pharmaceuticals as a medical treatment, there tends to be an equally strong side effect present as a spinoff. Because of this fact, the efficacy or risk/benefit ratio of any drug regimen becomes a fundamental issue in treatment decisions. In other words, does the supposed benefit of any particular treatment regimen warrant the risk of side effects known to accompany it? One doesn't want to be in the position where the cure is worse than the disease. To naturalists even the slightest risk of a side effect from a nonendogenous and nonnatural source is worrisome.

And justifiably so, as the true side effects of any specific drug action and interaction are never completely known. It is estimated that in the United States 60,000 to 140,000 people die per year from drug side effects and drug interactions.[4]

The mainstay of a more naturalistic physician's treatment protocol would be proper exercise, proper diet, added nutritive therapies, as well as any form of stress reduction by natural means. It is this belief structure that has led to the more recent usage of megavitamin therapy, first formulated by Linus Pauling, a Nobel laureate scientist who believed that high dose vitamin C would protect against the common cold.

While certainly this is not a mainstay belief of allopathic medical physicians, there is some significant research in large study populations (i.e., the Armed Forces) to indicate that both the severity and duration of the common cold are reduced by vitamin C.

In my own specialty of ophthalmology, there is a great deal of basic laboratory and early clinical research to show that antioxidant therapies as well as the addition of zinc, for instance, have a significant role to play in the overall metabolism of the eye.

The fundamental mechanism of megavitamin therapy is that a sick cell must expend a great deal of energy to transport waste products out of the cell and beneficial ions into the cell. By artificially changing the plasma gradient of the extracellular matrix through exogenous means, one can promote the natural ease of influx for advantageous ions into the cell with a minimum of energy expenditure by the cell.

While this is certainly not a mainstream scientific belief at present, I would predict that in the future much research will be done to determine a therapeutic window through which meganutrient therapy can be advantageous.

Another basic tenet of the naturalistic physician's belief is that Nature as a whole exists as a vibrant, self-sustaining, balanced organism and that man as part of this natural world should, in his pristine innocent state, exist in a natural balance himself. This, of course, sounds very reminiscent of the cultural beliefs of the American Indians with their close ties to the natural world and their belief structure that man exists in harmony with the natural world or else disharmony will arise within his life and culture.

Thus, the proper diet assumes extreme importance for maintaining one's balance in this natural state. Twenty-four years after its publication, Adelle Davis's book *Let's Eat Right to Keep Fit* is still of timely importance. This book is a well-documented report on the qualitative decline of the U.S. diet with the rise of industrialization. It also is a reflection of the decline in U.S. health associated with a poor industrialized diet. One might well conclude that the overfeeding of highly processed foods is the main cause for the epidemic diseases of the rich in Western civilization.[5] What we see in the health-food industry today is a backlash or return to more natural eating habits.

Perhaps the most extreme example of this is the discipline called macrobiotics. Macrobiotics is not a specific diet or nutritional program. It is, rather, a way of living that respects the physical, biological, emotional, mental, ecological, and spiritual order of our daily lives. It begins with the realization that there is a natural order to all things. Eating and living within this natural order leads to the promotion of health and happiness. The word *macrobiotics* comes from the Greek words *macro,* meaning large or great, and *bios,* meaning life.

While the principles of the macrobiotic diet go back several thousand years to ancient Oriental medicine, the first person to use the term *macrobiotics* was George Ohsawa (1893-1966). As a young man in Japan, he cured himself of tuberculosis with the macrobiotic diet. He recommended changing one's diet to low fat, low protein, high complex carbohydrate, and high fiber. According to his theory, man's foods in order of importance are grains, vegetables, salt, oil, nuts, fruits, and fish.

An important part of the macrobiotic philosophy is also that only locally grown produce normally in season locally is to be consumed. For example, if it is winter in Chicago, you would not eat squash (normally grown there only in the summer) even though it can be air-freighted in reasonably fresh condition.

Typically, whole cereal grains compose at least 50% by volume of every meal. These can include oats, barley, corn, millet, rye, wheat, and brown rice prepared in a variety of ways. Soups made with vegetables, grains, seaweed, or beans also comprise about 5% to 10% of daily food intake. Beans and sea vegetables comprise another 5% to 10%. Foods to avoid include meat, poultry, eggs, dairy products, animal fats, refined sugar, tropical and semitropical fruits, fruit juices, canned or frozen foods, coffee, tea, and nightshade vegetables (potatoes, tomatoes, peppers, and eggplant).[6]

Macrobiotics represents an extreme measure the patient can use to force his body to detoxify. The purity of this diet decreases the amount of energy necessary to process food. Theoretically, this resultant gain in energy promotes a natural detoxification of the body resulting in the improved health of the consumer.

It is of interest that many oncologists believe in the efficacy of a macrobiotic diet as an adjunct to orthodox Western oncologic therapies. This is because there is basic research to suggest that the usage of this modality provides a jolt to the immune system, which may trigger a natural healing response hitherto missing. Dr. Keith Block of Chicago, Illinois, is, perhaps, the prototype of how conventional physicians add complementary treatments to mainstream orthodox medicine. He is medical director of the cancer treatment program at an affiliate hospital of the University of Illinois and, additionally, is vice president of a Chicago chapter of the American Cancer Society. He has also done work for the advisory board of the Office of Technology Assessment Report on Unconventional Cancer Therapies for the U.S. Congress.

Dr. Block's treatment model consists of an advanced diet program with several innovative techniques that decrease the side effects of conventional therapies and enhance their effectiveness. Dr. Block originally developed his nutritional program by clinically modifying the macrobiotic regimen. An excellent review of his treatment program can be found in Chapter 17 of Michael Lerner's new book *Choices In Healing*.[7]

Dr. Block is not alone in his feelings regarding the importance of diet as adjuvant therapy. The American Cancer Society, National Cancer Institute, and American Institute for Cancer Research have all recommended what can be loosely called the "anticancer diet." These dietary guidelines are based on conclusions of the nation's leading experts who have carefully reviewed worldwide studies of eating habits . . . and the latest scientific evidence of the influence of diet and nutrition on the development of cancer.

Currently, the National Cancer Institute estimates that about one-third of all cancer deaths may be related to what a person eats over a long period of time. It is our present belief that cancer does not just suddenly appear, but rather develops very slowly through different stages, some of which are reversible. It may be that the type of food a person eats can affect many or perhaps all of these stages of development.

Diet and nutrition can work in two ways to help prevent cancer. The first is to avoid or consume only in moderation foods that are known to contain significant levels of carcinogens and foods that seem to provide the type of environment the cancer cells need for growth. The second is by consuming quantities of foods containing nutrients and other compounds that seem to stimulate the body's natural defense mechanisms and destroy carcinogens.[7]

The general dietary guidelines for the anticancer diet are:

1. Reduce the amount of fats consumed (especially saturated fats)

2. Reduce consumption of smoked and salt-and nitrate-cured foods (bacon; smoked ham, cheese, and seafood; corned beef, pastrami, and luncheon meats)

3. Eat high-fiber foods (whole grains, cereals, legumes, fruits, and vegetables)

4. Eat foods rich in vitamins A and C and beta carotene (dark green leafy vegetables, red, yellow, and orange vegetables and fruits, and citrus fruits and their juices)

5. Eat cruciferous vegetables (cabbage family)

6. Avoid or consume only in moderation alcoholic beverages.[8]

The concept of fasting is, likewise, an attempt to allow the system to detoxify. Even more extreme than a macrobiotic diet, one eliminates the energy used for digestion of food completely and, in theory, allows the body to detoxify as a result. Naturally, fasting is a more drastic option and should only be done under the guidance of an expert health-care professional in this field.

Finally, we reach the subject of dietary supplements. A basic assumption of the naturalistic physician and consumer who use dietary supplements is that within the natural world there already exists a set of

---

RATIONALE OF COMMONLY USED NUTRIENT/HERBAL SUPPLEMENTS

1) Vitamin A, C, E	➡ antioxidant properties
2) Turmeric	➡ antimutagenic, free radical scavenger, lowers cholesterol, affects platelet aggregation factor, anti-inflammatory
3) Bioflavanoids	➡ reduces capillary permeability, enhances utilization of ascorbic acid
4) Chlorella	➡ trace nutrient source, expecially of chlorophyll, contains respiratory, skin, and growth factor

chart continued on next page

continued from page 9

5) Melissa	⇥	calmative, digestive enhancer
6) Rosemary	⇥	antioxidant, digestive enhancer
7) Schizandrae Fruit	⇥	promotes natural physiological balance, increased vitality/energy
8) Royal Jelly	⇥	trace nutrient source
9) Barley Grass	⇥	rich in chlorophyll, trace minerals, amino acids; superoxide dismutase
10) Ginko Leaf	⇥	promotes cerebral vascular circulation
11) Ginger	⇥	enhances digestion, anti-inflammatory, antiparasitical, antibacterial
12) Siberian Ginseng	⇥	trace nutrient source
13) Horsetail Grass	⇥	source of silica, diuretic as synergistic to connective-tissue metabolism
14) Coriander	⇥	carminative
15) Dandelion Root	⇥	enhances liver detoxification
16) Nettle Leaf	⇥	trace nutrient source
17) Fennel Seed	⇥	carminative, respiratory emulsant
18) Spirulina Algae	⇥	rich in chlorophyll and beta-carotene, calcium, iron, and thicosimine
19) Chinese Ginseng	⇥	trace nutrient source
20) Hawthorne Leaf & Berry	⇥	circulatory enhancement as an iontrope
21) Aloe Vera	⇥	soothing, digestive enhancer, potential immune benefits
22) Artichoke Leaf	⇥	liver detoxification and regeneration
23) Saffron	⇥	trace nutrient source

24) Peppermint Oil	➤➤	enhances digestion
25) Anise Oil	➤➤	estrogenic agent/digestive enhancer
26) Lavender Oil	➤➤	promotes wound healing, enhances digestion, calming effect
27) Cinnamon	➤➤	carminative, antibacterial agent
28) Chamomile	➤➤	calming effect, enhances digestion, antibacterial, antiviral
29) Licorice Root	➤➤	antiviral, antiulcer, carminative
30) Sarsaparilla Root	➤➤	enhances liver detoxification
31) Green Oats	➤➤	aphrodisiac, counteracts nicotine addiction
32) Strawberry	➤➤	free radical scavenger, skin purifier
33) Papaya	➤➤	digestive enheancer, free radical scavenger
34) Pineapple	➤➤	digestive enhancer
35) Rice Bran	➤➤	fiber, anticholesterol [9, 10]

"super foods" or "super nutrients" that, if taken in a proper balance, will promote the natural harmony of the body, thereby resulting in a naturally healthy state.

On a molecular level one can consider these super foods as the amino acids, for instance. Vitamin levels, which although controversial at present, surely must be met at a certain minimum to ensure the proper functioning of the body itself. To the naturalist things such as chlorella, bee pollen, ginseng, ginger, algae and a host of other supplements exist to promote additional health advantages to the body.

A table has been prepared listing the basic beliefs that the consumer has regarding these food supplements and their motivation for using them.

Again, while I do not wish to debate the validity of any particular dietary supplement — and certainly large clinical trials in the traditional double-blind fashion are not abundant — there certainly exists a wealth of basic scientific research alluding to various potential benefits to the consumer.

3

Naturopathy

What is naturopathy? Naturopathy is a philosophy of disease elimination without drugs. According to its practitioners, it is based on the principle of cooperation with the natural laws governing all life in the universe. These biological laws control all of creation, from the planets rotating in space to the hormones circulating within our bodies. Naturopathy makes use of only natural agencies like water, air, light, heat, exercise, food, and electricity for the purposes of curing disease.

The naturopathic physician does not deny the modern advances made in biophysics, biochemistry, physiology, microbiology, and other investigational medical sciences. However, for the naturopathic physician these sciences only document the various processes taking place in the human body that can be healed naturally, either directly or indirectly, by adhering to this philosophy.

To the naturopathic physician, the cardinal principle that should govern every physician or other person who engages in the treatment of the sick should be to *act in harmony with nature.*

Naturopathy is a distinct system of treatment by itself. Although it may share common features, it is totally distinct from allopathy, Ayurveda (East Indian), homeopathy, etc.

Perhaps the first doctor historically to contribute to the early formation of the science of naturopathy was Hippocrates. Hippocrates, according to tradition, was born in 460 B.C. on the island of Cos off the shores of Asia Minor, near the Aesculapion, where his father was a priest. He was destined to become the greatest doctor of ancient Greece.

Hippocrates stressed two ways of preserving health and preventing disease: number one, by ensuring a healthy environment; number two, by healthy personal habits. The greatest contribution of Hippocrates was to stress the importance of preventative medicine as distinct from curative medicine and to point out the ancient truth that "prevention is better than cure."

Hippocrates was also the first to clearly delineate the cardinal rule of naturopathy, which is the following: "Nature is the healer of disease. Nature itself finds means and ways. The task of the physician is to help nature in any way he can, not to try to do too much himself, but to make it possible for nature to effect her cure."[1]

The naturalistic healing arts, which were prevalent in the Greek and Roman civilizations, subsequently were revived in modern times by Adolph Just, in 1896 when he presented his theory in the book *Return to Nature*. It was this book that so profoundly influenced Mahatma Gandhi that he not only adopted the "nature-cure" as his philosophy of life, but was also impelled to found a nature-cure center for the relief of the poor in the village of Uruli Kanchan, near Poona, where he himself acted as a physician.

To quote Adolph Just, "Who tells the children of Nature in distant countries, the animals of the woods how they are to bathe, what they are to eat, and how to avoid danger? The voices of Nature alone: instinct and the organs of sense (the sense of hearing, smelling, tasting, etc.) are their guides."[2]

Interestingly enough, Adolph Just lived to the ripe old age of ninety-eight years. This is rather remarkable considering that at fifty-two years of age he was in very poor health, until he developed and adopted for himself the system of naturopathy.

Yet it was Benedict Lust (1872-1945) who was credited with being the father of naturopathy. He graduated from the Universal Osteopathic

College of New York in 1898 and from the Eclectic Medical College of New York in 1913. Dr. Lust published many books throughout his career on topics as diverse as vitamin therapy, zone therapy, herbs and their uses, hot water therapies, and a universal naturopathic encyclopedia.

Unfortunately, he spent most of his life embattled with the more traditional Western medical societies who attempted to both professionally and politically disenfranchise his ideas and reputation.

For the practitioner of naturopathy, there is only one real cause of disease: "The one common cause of all disease is the presence of foreign substances in the body." The second main tenet is that: "Nature is the only curative agency."[3] We can assist nature only by removing the obstacles that prevent or retard its active operation.

According to the naturopathic physician, we best assist nature not by adding more impurities to the system, as is universally done in allopathic medicine, but by natural purificatory means only.

These natural purificatory means have been derived from observation of the animal kingdom:

> "Look to animals — wild, preferably — who live nearer to nature than does man, and see what animals do under such circumstances. In following them, we cannot go far wrong; and were we implicitly to follow the dictates of nature, there would be but little sickness in the world, and that little easily and rapidly cured.
>
> "Now what do animals do when they are diseased? If we observe them closely, we notice that they rest and sleep an unusual amount; that they drink a far greater quantity of water than they usually do; and that in cases of real sickness, they totally abstain from all food. This is invariably the case."[4]

According to the naturopathic doctor, the great laws of nature are never out of date. They are the same for all living beings. They are as true today as they were when first propounded 2,500 years ago. Fasting, proper diet, the correct use of air, light, rest, exercise, and bathing are all that is required for a successful cure — simply because these are the true, natural, and only real curative agencies in the universe. If this philosophy seems simplistic, that is exactly how it is meant to be perceived.

The second basic principle of naturopathy is called "the unity of disease." The principle of the unity of disease is that, regardless of the symptoms manifested and regardless of the name or names given to the symptoms or group of symptoms, it is one and the same thing in every case. In other words, all diseases have the same basis.

For the physician of naturopathy, the disease is caused by the body's inability to eliminate toxins successfully. It is their contention that a healthy body depends upon being regularly cleansed of poisonous waste material via the four eliminative channels (the skin, the lungs, the kidneys, and the bowels); should this system break down, disease thus ensues. It is further their belief that once this autointoxication takes place on a cellular level, then it manifests more grossly as various diseases or symptom complexes.

For the naturopathic physician, the patient who has eczema is merely exhibiting the accumulation of poison within his body that is so great that an unusual effort is being made to dispose of it through the skin.

A similar example is the patient who exudes a heavy accumulation of mucus from the nose and throat. This is merely a natural effort of the body to eliminate the overflow of toxins within it.

Another example is the patient with rheumatism. Physicians of naturopathy believe that this is an illustration of the way in which the body works to avoid injury to vital organs. If a system is so autointoxicated that no proper elimination of internal toxicity can occur, it is then deposited in muscles or joints as a natural protective mechanism of avoiding more vital organs, such as the heart. When important vital organs are finally involved, no further help can be given to the patient, and death ensues.

Clearly, in this scientific age the naturopathic physician would not deny the existence of infectious agents as a part of the disease process. Their contention, rather, is that the infectious agent is not the primary etiological cause, but once again only a symptom of the system's imbalance. The (systems) in efficient functioning has created a seat in which the infectious agent is then able to invade and occupy. It is their belief that faulty living, unhygienic surroundings, and wrong mental and emotional states impair the vital functions of the body, causing a disturbance of the chemical actions and reactions or faulty metabolism.

According to naturopathic philosophy, metabolic disturbance

leads to a breakdown in the protective mechanisms of the normal bacteriologic flora. It is the loss of the proper balance of beneficent to virulent bacteria in the digestive tract that signals the first stage of the disease process. Once this imbalance has occurred, an ever worsening spiral of autotoxicity creating disease manifestation then ensues. As the proper elimination of waste products breaks down, the chemical imbalance found in the physiology continues to worsen. This process will continue to spiral until the naturopathic physician intervenes by setting up the proper conditions for the body to naturally purify and relieve itself of the accumulated toxins.

It is interesting to note that, despite their "naturalness," homeopathic remedies are no more accepted by the naturopathic physician than allopathic pharmaceuticals. Both pharmaceuticals and homeopathy have sought to restore health by producing (in some sense mimicking) disease. "They have employed, as the proper agents to restore health to the sick, those things that are known to produce sickness in those who are well. Indeed, how can any natural-cure practitioner subscribe to the principle of restoring health by measures that impair health?"[5]

It may seem unusual that to the naturopathic physician the ability to arrive at a correct diagnosis is not as important as the ability to aid the body in its natural healing function. It is the belief of naturaopaths that modern medicine is much too concerned with the naming of disease and too little concerned with the cause and prevention of the trouble.

To summarize this philosophy:

> "All disease is one. The multifacets and different symptoms are merely the body's effort to cleanse itself of the accumulated surfeit effete matter — the one cause of all disease. The effete or foreign matter accumulates due to faulty elimination of the body wastes or due to invasion from outside of living or nonliving material or both on account of faulty habits of living [by the patient]. The symptoms differ because of the differing forms of foreign matter that acts as a stimulus to the disease process. As the disease is one and the cause is one, so the treatment is one — almost similar for all cases — example fasting, eliminative and building diet, exercise, massage

and other natural methods, and structural adjustments to help nature in its eliminative cleansing process. Fasting helps to clean out quickly. Fasting also suppresses infection as nothing else does. Drugs and medicines and poisons of whatever school or kind have no place innate in 'nature cure.' They all produce undesirable side effects, and add more foreign matter, thereby perpetuating disease instead of curing it.[6]

4

Homeopathy

Homeopathy is perhaps the most confusing of all alternative medical-care systems in that it has definite origins in traditional Western medicine. Despite this common origin, however, its usage varies greatly depending upon the continent involved.

Homeopathy is extremely common in Europe, particularly in Germany and France where it is very popular. In the United Kingdom it has always been available under the National Health Service. There currently exist six homeopathic hospitals, including the Royal London Homeopathic Hospital, in the United Kingdom, where homeopathic remedies are used along with the standard drugs.

In Russia there is a system of polyclinics, notably in Moscow and St. Petersburg, which specialize in homeopathic treatments. Homeopathy is also officially recognized as a specialty in Brazil and India.[1]

However, in the United States the use of homeopathy has been far less widespread. The number of active practitioners is relatively small compared to the number of general allopathic physicians.

What Is This Unusual Science?

Homeopathy is a form of complimentary medicine, which relies heavily on observation and experience. The three distinguishing characteristics of homeopathy are that:

1. remedies are prescribed based on the totality of a person's symptoms

2. that the remedy likely to cure a person is a dilution of that substance which would cause the same symptoms in a healthy person

3. that the remedies are prepared using microdoses of substances, which are diluted and then vigorously shaken.

Homeopathy was the discovery of a German physician, Samuel Hahnemann (1755-1843). A precociously brilliant man, he had mastered eight languages and turned himself into an outstanding experimental chemist by the time he obtained his medical degree in 1799.

He had followed the orthodox training of the day with its insistence on powerful drugging, bleeding, and blistering; but he soon grew first disillusioned, then appalled by the failure of these methods in practice. Far from curing his patients, he felt he was becoming a "murderer or a malefactor,"[2] a thought so terrible to him that he gave up practice and concentrated on his chemical work and his writings.

In his wide reading, Hahnemann had previously come across the medical theory that "like cures like." It is common in German folk medicine and is also found in Greek medical writings.

Hahnemann soon tested this theory by dosing himself with cinchona regularly for several days. Cinchona (a Peruvian bark that yields quinine) at that time was the specific cure for malaria. Hahnemann noticed that by dosing himself he brought on all the symptoms classic for malaria, including intermittent fevers. These rapidly subsided when he stopped taking the drug.

Other drugs, he reasoned, might be used in the same way once their action in a healthy person had been determined. To establish this new science, Hahnemann, by this time a professor at Leipzig University in Germany, instituted a series of experimental studies with a chosen band of students. He called these studies his "provings."

Over a period of time, this group dosed themselves with particular drugs and made elaborately detailed notes of their reactions: physical, emotional, and mental. To define his new science, Hahnemann coined the term "Similis similbus curentur"— Let like be cured by like. This means that a substance capable of producing a certain set of symptoms in a healthy person will, when taken in a minute, specially prepared, form . . . cure a similar set of symptoms exhibited by someone who is already sick.

In contrast to the allopathic view, where the symptoms of disease constitute the entire problem in itself, the homeopathic perspective sees symptoms as a unified effort made by the individual's constitution to return to a state of health and well being. Therefore, any momentum the homeopathic physician can provide to the symptomatology is enhancing the body's own natural mechanisms of self-cure.

The homeopathic remedy acts as a stimulus or catalyst to the curative powers of the patient's own constitution. For example, homeopathic thinking would interpret the symptom of diarrhea as a condition of the body trying to eliminate waste from itself in order to get better. The proper homeopathic intervention, therefore, would be to administer a tiny dose of a substance that, in a crude form, would cause diarrhea in order to assist and resolve this process. This is diametrically opposed to the manner in which most allopathic physicians would treat diarrhea, which is to arrest it altogether.

When Dr. Hahnemann began testing this theory, he found it succeeded in bringing about a more holistic cure to the patient. And, in the process, he made yet another discovery, again almost by accident: The smaller the dose, the more effective it is. He began diluting his drugs more and more, until he was in effect administering a medicine in which not a molecule of the original substance remained.

A good example of a homeopathic remedy is the extract belladonna. This is derived from a highly poisonous plant known as deadly night-shade. Conventional physicians prescribe drops of tincture of belladonna for a variety of gastrointestinal problems, but homeopaths use belladonna in even smaller dilutions. The dosage that homeopathic physicians commonly use for problems such as croup in children or bronchitis in adults is know as 30C. The "C" stands for a 1 in 100 dilution. That means that one drop of belladonna extract is dissolved in 99 drops of water/alcohol solution, then one drop of the new solution is further diluted by 99 drops of liquid, and so on, thirty times. After thirty dilutions the concentration of belladonna would be expressed scientifically as 1 over 10 to the 60th.

According to the laws of chemistry and probability, a remedy that has been prepared at a *10 to the 24th* dilution — that is, a homeopathic dosage of 12C — would theoretically be diluted just past the point where a dose contains a single molecule of the original substance. At the greater dilutions, which are often used in homeopathy, the odds that there could be any of the original active substance left at all decrease almost to zero.

While the mechanism by which these medicines work seems almost mystical, homeopaths use the analogy of vaccination as an example of an orthodox application of Hahnemann's discovery. Desensitization therapy by an allergist is also analogous to their treatment philosophy.

From his experimental studies, Hahnemann gradually built up a collection of about ninety-nine remedies. Some were taken from minerals, such as arsenic and sulfur, some from animals (the most famous of which is lachesis, taken from the venom of a particularly deadly tropical snake).

Interestingly, he found that however poisonous in normal doses the action of a drug, it was therapeutic in minute doses.

This coincides with a basic biological law formulated by two German scientists, Rudolph Arndt and Hugo Schultz. After repeated experiments they established that for poisonous substances, large doses kill, moderate doses paralyze, and small doses stimulate.

Even more interesting, Dr. Hahnemann also discovered that at a certain degree of dilution, the characteristic healing effect of a plant disappeared, to be replaced by a totally different action. The best example is that a homeopathic dose of opium might be given to arouse a near comatose patient.

While all this may be most puzzling to a mechanistic scientist, clearly the science of immunology has today established beyond all doubt that the human body has marvelous and elaborate defense mechanisms that are activated by an alien substance, be it infectious agent or drug. Perhaps these microdoses of alien substances are triggering the body's inherent mechanisms to promote a self-cure.

The French scientist Jacques Benveniste believed he had found such a mechanism experimentally when he published in June 1988 an article in the highly respected scientific journal *Nature*. His team reported that dilutions up to ten to a hundred-twentieth over it of an antibody (a substance produced by the immune system in response to infection) could evoke a reaction from a certain type of white blood cell. The research was confirmed in other laboratories, and *Nature*'s reviewers were unable to find a flaw that would invalidate the startling results. This publication created an international controversy, which to this day is unfinished.

Despite Hahnemann's failure to explain on a molecular level the ability of his dilutions to heal, by 1813 homeopathy had become a force to be reckoned with in Germany. Homeopaths were highly successful at treating the typhoid fever that Napoleon's tattered remnant of an army brought back with them from Moscow. And slowly, news of Hahnemann's theory spread throughout Europe, attracting many doctors who were dissatisfied, as he had been, with the medical practice of the day.

Among these was a young Danish medical student, Hans B. Gram, who opened North America's first homeopathic practice in New York City in 1825. Three years later one of his students, John F. Gray, opened a second.

By 1844 the homeopaths had united in New York to found the American Institute of Homeopathy. In Philadelphia the Hahnemann Medical College was turning out numbers of graduates educated to the very highest standards of the day. In 1900 there were more than twenty homeopathic colleges in the United States. However, by 1923 only two remained.

The decline of homeopathy was not accidental, but rather was a direct aim of a new organization — the American Medical Association (AMA). Much of the energies of this new organization in its formative years were directed toward discouraging the continued growth and success of homeopathy.

Despite this organized opposition, the success of homeopathy is not hard to understand historically. The homeopaths offered their patients not merely the charm of a novel medical theory, but almost the only painless therapy available. Regular allopathic physicians in the early 19th century were still utilizing bleeding, blistering, and drastic purging.[3]

Perhaps Oliver Wendell Holmes, addressing the Massachusetts Medical Society in 1860, sums up the mood of the day perfectly: "Apart from opium and a small number of specific drugs . . . I firmly believe that if the whole materia medica, as now used, could be sunk to the bottom of the sea, it would be all the better for mankind — and all the worse for the fishes."[4]

Given the competition of the day, homeopathy continued to be a huge success. By 1890, when the American Homeopathic Institute raised a monument to Dr. Hahnemann, the homeopathic physicians, in contrast to their allopathic counterparts, were clearly the wealthier, more successful, and enjoyed a higher status in the general populous.[5]

From what we have discussed already, it should be obvious that the basic assumption underlying homeopathy is that human beings have an internal homeostatic mechanism enabling them to interact comfortably with the environment most of the time. When a person's homeostasis is compromised in some serious way — by exposure to a very strong disease agent or allergen, by stress, by exhaustion, by ingestion of a toxic substance — the person becomes ill and manifests symptoms.

Homeopaths believe that the particular constellation of a person's symptoms is the key to prescribing a remedy for that person, since symptoms are the body's way of manifesting the conflict between its natural homeostasis and the interfering agent. Therefore, two persons with the same disease (according to the categories of orthodox Western medicine) but with different symptoms will be given different remedies by the homeopathic physician.

The examination of the patient as to symptomatology, therefore, becomes primary for the homeopathic physician. Given the importance of the patient's history, typically the first consultation takes about one and a half hours, then follow up sessions are usually forty-five minutes. During the initial history-taking session, the patient will be asked many questions: Initially these questions will focus around the presenting complaint. For example, if a person were suffering from migraines, the homeopath would need to know when they started, what was happening in the person's life during this period, how often the person gets them, what time of day they might occur, what factors affect the symptoms, the quality of the pain, etc.

In order to find a remedy that may be prescribed holistically, however, the homeopathic physician will also ask questions that focus on many other aspects of the person. These questions would include insights into the patient's personality, emotional makeup, relationship with the environment, and both the individual's own and the family medical history.

The task of the homeopath is to match a particular set of symptoms and character traits to those produced by a "remedy proving." In this fashion, each remedy can be considered to be tailor-made for an individual and his or her set of symptoms. For example, it is possible to have ten cases of influenza (which may all be of the same exact strain according to ortho-dox microbiology), each of which would require a different remedy as a result of a particular set of symptoms exhibited by each patient. Converse-ly, it is also possible to have ten completely different and unrelated illnesses that, after careful differentiation of symptoms, all require the same remedy.

This may be counterintuitive to the orthodox Western physician who places primary importance on naming the particular disease entity. But not so for homeopathy. Classical homeopathy believes in a hierarchy of symptomatology and that the treatment will be most effective when greater emphasis is placed on those symptoms and traits that occur at the mental and emotional plane as opposed to those symptoms manifested at the physical level. This does not mean physical symptoms are not con-sidered as important as mental or emotional complaints. Rather, it was discovered that remedies matching an individual's character makeup tend to be more effective in bringing about the cure of the whole person as opposed to remedies matched primarily to physical symptoms.

Homeopathic physicians do rely to some extent on the results of lab-oratory tests and on their own physical examination, but the patient's symptoms are still the most important source of information for their diagnosis and treatment.

Mainstream medicine criticizes homeopathy by saying that its gentle-ness has outlived its usefulness and that treatment successes are probably no more than placebo action. Homeopaths would counterargue that mul-tiple randomized, double-blinded, placebo-controlled studies have docu-mented the efficacy of homeopathic remedies beyond that of placebo. Furthermore, homeopaths would point out that their remedies work in children as well as animals, two patient groups usually thought to be resis-tant to placebos.[6,7,8,9]

Like most alternative health-care systems, the main objection of homeopathic physicians to mainstream allopathic medicine is that they feel the use of traditional pharmaceuticals is dangerous. These physi-cians prefer a more natural intervention, which has much less risk of upsetting the homeostasis of the physiology due to harsh side effects.

Perhaps the greatest stumbling block to homeopathy is the fact that de-spite clinical trials showing, in some series, that homeopathy works, there has not been an adequate explanation of the mechanisms of its action.[10]

To explain the action of homeopathic drugs according to basic pharmaceutical theories would be difficult. The process for making a homeopathic medicine involves serial dilutions in a proportion of one to nine or one to ninety-nine with vigorous shaking of the solution between dilutions. Surprisingly, the more dilutions, the higher the potency (according to homeopathic physicians). Some preparations, however, are so dilute that it is unlikely that a single molecule of the original substance is left in the medicine. This is because they have been diluted beyond Avogadro's number, which is the number of molecules in a mole of any particular substance.

Even if one were to grant that it is conceivable in lower potencies that these medicines have some pharmacological effect, it is incredible to the Western-trained physician that these higher potencies (greater dilutions) could work at all.

An interesting caveat to the story is that there is some evidence that vigorous shaking is crucial to the activity of homeopathic preparations. Clinical trials have shown that a preparation that has been diluted with vigorous shaking is effective, whereas the same preparation created by dilution only and not vigorously shaken is not effective clinically.[11] This is surprising considering that the mathematical concentration of the primary active substance is the same.

It is possible that the homeopathic physicians are correct in their belief that some sort of energy is imparted from the substance to the solvent. In other words, the medium, in a sense, becomes the message. In 1983 a study using magnetic resonance imaging showed that homeopathic remedies had distinctive readings of subatomic activity compared to placebo.[12]

Yet we remain a long way from explaining the mechanism of action on a molecular level for these remedies.

It is very possible that homeopathy, like many other alternative health-care systems (such as the traditional Chinese medical system), functions not on a chemical level of therapy but on an energy level of therapy.[13] Clearly, attempts at explaining the mechanism of action on a chemical basis are difficult to imagine. However, when one realizes the efficacy of acupuncture (aside from its endorphin stimulation) is solely based on an energy meridian theory, one can question whether homeopathy treats patients on the same level. Later chapters review acupuncture theory and practice and the philosophy of healing through the use of energy manipulation in more detail.

5

Herbal Medicines

The use of herbal medicines, as opposed to modern allopathic pharmaceuticals, is a mainstay of the ancient systems of medicine. Both the Chinese system of medicine, and the East Indian system of medicine, called Ayurveda, rely heavily on herbal medicines as a treatment option.

This should come as no surprise to modern pharmaceutical companies, as they readily utilize the basic folklore of more "primitive" native cultures worldwide as a source of potential leads for pharmaceutical development in the modern era.

It is well known, based on survey data from United States pharmacies, that 25% of all prescriptions dispensed from community pharmacies during the period 1962 to 1973 contained at least one active constituent still extracted from plant sources (not synthesized).[1] A common example often quoted in medical schools is the use of the drug Digitalis or digoxin for cardiac care, which derives from a common garden plant — foxglove.

Other plant-derived drugs commonly used today include atropine, codeine, ephedrine, leurocristine, morphine, pilocarpine, pseudoephedrine, quinidine, quinine, scopolamine, tubocurarine, and vincaleukoblastine. Indeed, these are the prototype drugs discussed in all pharmacology textbooks.

Many nonaccredited naturalistic schools of medicine exist teaching herbal medicine at this time. They include the California School of Herbal Studies and the School of Natural Healing in Park City, Utah. Operating alongside them are the accredited schools, such as John Bastyr College in Seattle and the National College of Naturopathic Medicine in Portland, Oregon. Both of these colleges are four-year, postgraduate schools with admission requirements comparable to those of conventional medical schools.

Books on herbal remedies abound in the bookstore as well as in Grandma's kitchen, especially among ethnic cultures in this country. They have woven their way into the basic fabric of our life in the resurgence of noncaffeinated herbal teas, readily available at many fine restaurants.

In health-food stores the consumer is provided with an array of common herbal treatments for routine ailments. Examples of these are the use of slippery elm in teas to combat the congestion of upper respiratory infections or the use of menthol teas to do the same.

The chart below lists some of the common herbal teas available in the market and their supposed mechanisms of action for common ailments:

- Chamomile — soothing, alleviates stress and insomnia
- Peppermint — helps indigestion, reduces fever, eases migraines
- Raspberry — aids sore throats and menstrual cramps
- Eucalyptus — improves breathing, helps clear chest infections
- Chrysanthemum — alleviates colds, detoxification
- Genmaicha — focuses and calms the mind
- Senna Leaf — laxative
- Licorice Root — soothing to throat mucosa

Modern herbalists maintain that plants are not only the safest way to administer medicine, but also the most effective. They point out that apart from their active principle, plants contain other substances that may enhance their therapeutic actions or reinforce the healing powers by a synergistic process not always fully understood. Digitalis provides a perfect example of both phenomena: Digitoxin and verodoxin are both glycocides found in foxglove; but unlike digitoxin, verodoxin on its own is valueless as a tonic for the heart. Add four parts of useless verodoxin to six parts of digitoxin (which does have a tonic action) and the resulting mix will have the same therapeutic effect as ten parts of digitoxin. Moreover, the brew will be less toxic than ten parts of digitoxin alone.[2]

There is also evidence to support another strongly held belief of herbalists — that extracted active principles on their own, lacking these built-in safety factors, may be substances much too potent for the human body to deal with. Dr. Alec Forbes, a physician who has become one of the strongest advocates of alternative therapies within the ranks of allopathy, mentions *rauvolfia* as an example. It has been in use for thousands of years in Ayurveda as a sedative. Mahatma Gandhi used to drink rauvolfia tea as a nightcap. Yet it has taken only twenty years for its most active alkaloid, reserpine, used in isolation, to go out of fashion because, although good for lowering blood pressure and sedation, it can cause severe depression.[3]

Pharmacologists will concede the relative safety of the whole plant as opposed to isolated chemical compounds because this is a difference they can measure by fairly simple toxicity testing in animals or humans.

The true herbalist, however, believes that the whole plant is both safer and more effective medicine than isolated bits of it or man-made chemical compounds that mimic it. Even more heretical to the modern scientific mind is the herbalist's suggestion that there could actually be any difference between a chemical compound extracted from a plant and the same chemical structure created synthetically in the laboratory out of coal-tar. According to classical biochemistry, the two are chemically identical, and there should be no difference.

An example to the contrary is the cinchona plant, traditionally used by Peruvian Indians as a cure for fevers; it was first brought to the West by Jesuit priests in 1739. From it was isolated quinine — the best-known cure for malaria. A synthetic version was created in the 1940s, when World War II cut off supplies from the main production area of the East Indies, where it had been smuggled and introduced by the Dutch in the 1800s. To this day, however, the natural product is considered superior to all substitutes: Malaria can build up a resistance to the synthetics, but not to the genuine drug.[4]

Whether or not we accept that there is a biological distinction to be made between man-made chemicals on the one hand and the medicine extracted from a living plant on the other, the human body often behaves as though there is. The terrible toll of side effects from chemical medicines is the most eloquent argument possible that such a distinction can legitimately be made.

In fact, if herbal medicine does have one indisputable advantage in safety over chemical medicine, it is the fact that almost all of its drugs have been in clinical use for centuries of recorded use. History has provided doctors with longitudinal data to monitor any potential side effects.

This becomes increasingly important when we realize that according to the GAO (general accounting agency of the federal government), over 50% of all drugs approved by the FDA are later found to have extremely serious or even fatal side effects that were not gleaned during the pretesting phase of their scrutiny.[5] By contrast, it seems reasonable to assume that any plant drug with a centuries-long reputation for being perfectly safe as well as effective has probably earned that reputation.

Nonetheless, this is certainly not the stance taken by the federal government and the FDA:

> *"The American public does not have the knowledge*
> *to make wise health-care decisions. . . . Trust us. We*
> *will tell you what is good for you. . . ."*[6]

Unfortunately, that is clearly not the case. Considering that "three of the top four causes of lethal poisonings in the U.S. are FDA-approved drugs" and that a toxicity category is virtually nonexistent for herbal dietary supplements, it seems irrational that the FDA is bent on the regulation of the health-food industry with such zeal.[7]

In fact, the FDA's "war" to regulate virtually all traditional medicine or tonic herbs out of the U.S. marketplace is truly a threat to both national health and medical freedom of choice:

> "Some so-called dietary-supplement products
> that have no recognized nutritional role are sold
> for therapeutic uses. It is a simple fact that these
> products (herbs) are legally drugs and should be
> properly regulated as such," said Michael R. Tay-
> lor, FDA Deputy Commissioner of Policy.[8]

One can clearly see the tension that currently exists between governmental control exercised through the arm of the FDA versus the interests of the alternative health-care consumer to re-empower himself. As Ivan Illich reminds us in his concept of a "radical monopoly," radical monopolies do more than disable people from doing or making things on their own. They impinge still further on freedom and independence. The ultimate disservice is when it turns mutual care and self-medication into misdemeanors and felonies.[9]

As we shall see later in our chapter on challenges to the future, there exists an unholy alliance between the FDA and the pharmaceutical industry, which will make progress to adopt a more rational health-care system very difficult. We will explore this alliance in more detail.

6

Chiropractic/Massage

Daniel David Palmer was the founder of chiropractic in the late nineteenth century. According to historical accounts, Dr. Palmer heard a patient complaining that he had lost his hearing years before when he bent over and something "went" in his back. Palmer discovered a misplaced vertebra in the man's back and by careful manipulation locked it back into place. Needless to say, the man recovered his hearing shortly afterward.

Dr. Palmer's earliest belief was that the subluxation of individual vertebrae was the cause of all disease. Even minor derangements, bad posture, or inflammation can cause defective working of the nerves passing up the hollow center of the cord, with widely disparate results such as the deafness that Palmer described in his first case.

Dr. Palmer opened the first chiropractic school in Davenport, Iowa, in 1897. Named the National School of Chiropractic, it was moved to Chicago in 1908, where it was headed by John A. Howard.

Dr. Howard developed a more expanded view of chiropractic, believing "innervation by adjustment often is not sufficient. We must aid nature

in a natural and congenital manner . . . eliminate accumulated waste . . .
stop autotoxemia . . . balance the diet . . . relieve constipation . . . and in
practice there are so many conditions to meet, pathological tissue changes
to overcome which are beyond the reach of spinal technic that to claim 'no
limitations' for a simple technique is beyond the scope of truth or reason."[1]

By strict definition chiropractic is a hands-on, drugless, nonsurgical
form of health care. In Greek the derivation of the word *chiropractic*
comes from "cheir," meaning hand, and "praktitos," meaning to do. So
quite literally, chiropractic is that which is practiced or done by hand.

More than 125 chiropractic colleges have been opened since 1897.
However, the vast majority have undergone mergers among themselves
or have simply gone out of business. Currently fourteen colleges of chiropractic exist in seven states.

An offshoot of chiropractic occurred in 1905 when Oakley Smith,
an 1899 graduate of the Palmer School of Chiropractic, founded naprapathy. In contrast to Dr. Palmer's belief in the subluxation theory of disease, Dr. Smith believed that scarring and subsequent shortening of the
soft connective tissue supporting the human skeleton was the causative
effect responsible for the structural irregularities of the joints and subsequent neurovascular interference. Practitioners of naprapathy thus concern themselves with the manipulation of the soft connective tissues
rather than the actual bony vertebrae themselves.

It is difficult for the allopathic Western physician to believe that all
disease processes stem from such a simple, isolated explanation of the
body's pathology. And the fact that mainstream medicine was more or
less outraged at this simplistic notion of disease and the claims made
thereof was not lost on the founders of chiropractic.

The official catalogue of the National College of Chiropractic from
the years 1918 through 1930 carried this disclaimer: "This school holds
that there is so much good in chiropractic that the ridiculous and exor-
bitant claims often advanced by poorly trained chiropractors do their
profession more harm than good. Our aim is toward rationalism, not
radicalism."[2]

Nonetheless, the very existence of chiropractic as an alternative
medical therapy spurred what can only be construed as a "cold war"
between mainstream allopathic medicine and chiropractic. Chiropractors historically claim that this cold war was sustained by propaganda

based upon intellectual dishonesty, fear, avarice, and professional jealousy. This historic contest was finally put to rest in 1987, after an eleven-year court battle, when a federal judge ruled that the AMA and two other medical groups had broken antitrust laws by engaging in a long-standing campaign to "contain and eliminate chiropractic." Today chiropractic represents the third-largest group of health-care professionals (behind physicians and dentists, who are first and second respectively) with 50,000 licensed chiropractors.

It may surprise the current medical student to know that as late as 1960 the code of ethics of the American Medical Association (AMA) continued to classify "all voluntary associations with chiropractors, osteopaths, and optometrists as unethical."[3]

There is no doubt that chiropractic historically developed in order to fill a void in the current practice of medicine. As medicine became more technological and subspecialized, the change from a hands-on physician to a hands-off physician was dramatic. Thus a vacuum developed whereby the effects of true human touch and its relationship to the nature of healing was lost.

Chiropractors and their colleagues, such as naprapaths, represent the major entry point of the consumer into the alternative health-care medical establishment. As we've discussed, chiropractic schools vary widely in both their belief system as to the primacy of one technique over another as well as in their practical application (i.e., manipulations).

I, personally, have been to a variety of chiropractors for treatment of various ailments and can attest to the wide discrepancies in their skill levels, efficacy levels, and safety levels. As with all health-care professionals, allopathic physicians included, skills and treatment successes vary according to the individual.

My own preference is for chiropractic schools that promote a very gentle type of manipulation, allowing the natural mechanisms of the body to spontaneously "realign" after stimulation by an external impetus. I have been successfully cured from years of chronic debilitating low back pain and sciatica by very minor manipulations combined with acupuncture.

Chiropractors as a group use perhaps the widest variety of treatment modalities that exist. Depending on the school and orientation of the individual practitioner, they may weight their treatment protocol heavily toward a Chinese or Indian type of philosophy using pulse diagnosis and/or acupuncture. Other chiropractors manipulate the physiology through herbal medicines or meganutrient therapy.

Early in their history, chiropractors split into two camps, the "straights" and "mixers." The straights were inspired by Palmer's admonition to keep chiropractic "pure, straight, and unadulterated." The straights hold close to their master's original beliefs and favor manipulation as their therapeutic mainstay. The mixers, on the other hand, are more likely to look beyond classical chiropractic by making a medical diagnosis, collaborating with M.D.s, and adding such ancillary therapies as ultrasound, massage, electrical stimulation, acupuncture, homeopathy, or herbal medicines.

An interesting diagnostic tool found exclusively in the chiropractic field is that of applied kinesiology. Applied kinesiology is a technique that utilizes muscle testing to determine the appropriateness of a treatment regimen for an individual patient. In practice, a patient would lie flat, for instance, and have a treatment regimen placed on his navel or surrounding area. The practitioner would then test the strength of one's muscular response to this regimen, similar to muscle-strength testing during a rudimentary neurology examination.

By gauging the active resistance of a set muscle group both before and after the exogenous substance is placed close to the body, practitioners believe they can document the future efficacy or harmonious potential of this new treatment agent for the individual patient.

Although I do not use applied kinesiology as a diagnostic modality in my own professional practice, I have personally experienced it as a patient and marveled at its repeatability. Thus, it certainly appears not to be a figment of imagination of either the practitioner or consumer that this type of testing can be done. Whether it can predict the success of any given treatment regimen for an individual patient, is a far more complex issue.

The empiric success of applied kinesiology requires a more subtle level or basis by which it can be explained. By the use of the term "more subtle basis," I am referring to the concept of an energy field surrounding the more physical manifestation of our bodies as we generally know them.

It should come as no surprise to anyone familiar with modern science that an energy field must certainly exist surrounding a living body, since all living organisms exhibit a certain manifestation of energy and in fact are defined as "living" by that special quality of energy we know as life itself.

In the recent era many investigators of parapsychology as well as other related health-care fields have been interested in the documentation of this energy field by such techniques as Kirlian photography. Kirlian photography purports to document the various states of an energy field as it exists around a human being. Developed by Semyon Kirlian in Russia, this special process records on film the corona discharge, or aura, of an object/subject.

Perhaps a more mainstream way to think of this is the use of thermal imaging, which can demonstrate blood flow throughout the body. This also is a definite form of energy field, although it is thermal in nature and not magnetic. It is the fluctuation of this energy field that purportedly lies at the basis of techniques such as applied kinesiology.

There is no doubt that back pain is a major health-care issue costing the country billions annually in medical expenses and lost work time. According to surveys, back pain affects more than three-quarters of us during our lifetime; it second only to the common cold as a reason for office visits and second only to childbirth as a reason for hospitalization. There is little doubt that manipulation can be very beneficial for most forms of acute back pain.

In 1993 the Ontario Ministry of Health issued a report specifically about the value of manipulation in the management of low-back pain. This was known as the Manga Report for its lead author, economist Pran Manga. The report stated that chiropractic manipulation is safer, more effective, and more cost-effective than medical management of low-back pain.

Dr. Paul G. Shekelle, an internist who headed the Rand Corporation project to review published research on manipulation, also agrees. Though the body of research on low-back pain supports spinal manipulation, not chiropractic per se, "A good chiropractor will give a better exam and better advice and treatment than an average internist or family physician. The general practitioner doesn't feel comfortable with back pain. He'll give the patient Tylenol and send him home to bed."[4]

While chiropractors may have found their niche in treating low-back pain by spinal manipulation, they have both a credibility and a liability issue with many members of the American public as well as the scientific community. The credibility issue surrounds the fact that besides manipulation, chiropractors may use unorthodox forms of nutritional counseling, claiming that the use of vitamins, minerals, and food supplements can treat or prevent disease. While much basic research may point in this direction, certainly double blinded, randomized, controlled studies have not been done in most cases.

In a survey published last year by the National Board of Chiropractic Examiners, 84% of chiropractors responded that they had used "nutritional counseling therapy or supplements." The same survey found that 37% of chiropractors use homeopathic remedies and applied kinesiology as a diagnostic tool.

A great deal of skepticism arises because the mechanism of action for most chiropractic treatments cannot be scientifically elucidated, much like the remedies in homeopathy. In Dr. Palmer's day, when the age of medicine had just begun, his theory of chiropractic was a reasonable conjecture to understand the mysteries of health and disease. But now, a century later, it is clear that the nervous system is not the "master of all bodily functions." For example, a person who is quadriplegic retains normal function of most internal organs, despite massive injury to the spinal cord. Other critical nerves (such as the cranial nerves) affecting face, eyes, ears, tongue, and throat also bypass the spine and are not amenable to spinal manipulation.

Chiropractic has had its share over the years of derogatory publicity. A major investigation published in 1975 by *Consumer Reports* found that chiropractors were likely to take unnecessary X-rays, perform manipulation on infants and children, propose inordinately lengthy treatment plans, and promote chiropractic treatment for serious disorders that needed medical care.

A report in 1986 from the U.S. Department of Health & Human Services Office of the Inspector General also showed that many chiropractors had been using excessive X-rays in an effort to obtain Medicare reimbursement. Since Medicare coverage for chiropractic services was limited to the treatment of subluxations "demonstrated by X-ray to exist," a huge number of unnecessary X-rays were performed on unsuspecting patients. This is indefensible in light of the fact that

84% of chiropractors surveyed admitted that some subluxations don't show up on X-ray.

But chiropractic's liability issues run much deeper. Complications of manipulation can range from increased pain to ruptured disks, paralysis, and even death. The most serious injuries stem from manipulation of the neck, where damage to the arteries bringing blood to the brain can result in a stroke or other neurological problem. While it seems that only a handful of strokes have resulted from the many millions of manipulations done each year, the statistics may be misleading. In a literature search published by the *Journal of Neurosurgery* in 1992, only 1,112 published case reports of complications due to manipulation were found over a span of sixty-five years.

And while these statistics may appear safe initially, *Consumer Reports* cites figures derived from a prominent company providing malpractice insurance to U.S. chiropractors giving a much more alarming picture. According to *Consumer Reports*, in 1990 alone the company paid approximately 140 claims to patients who suffered a stroke after spinal manipulation. They also point out that the statistic may under-estimate the problem, as research shows that only a small fraction of patients who are injured through medical negligence ever file malpractice claims.[5]

While the problems surrounding chiropractic philosophy still exist today, an attempt at reform from within the profession has been made. Ten years ago a small group of chiropractors formed the National Association for Chiropractic Medicine and publicly renounced chiropractic philosophy. These members agreed to use manipulation as an applied science and to treat only neuromusculoskeletal conditions.

This year the association also added the word "orthopractic" at the end of its name to show its affiliation with the Orthopractic Manipulation Society International. This is a new organization made up of medical doctors, osteopaths, physical therapists, and chiropractors. The orthopractic guidelines define manipulation as a therapy for joints that lack adequate mobility and range of motion, not as a treatment for "mysterious" subluxations. The group has repudiated many practices associated with chiropractors; such as, full spine X-rays, the use of manipulation to treat postural disorders in children, infectious diseases, and internal and metabolic disorders. While orthopractic practitioners are still only a small part of the chiropractic community, they represent a credible alternative that may allow chiropractic to become embraced more easily by mainstream medicine.

An alternative also open to the referring medical doctor is to seek out certified physical therapists who typically are on staff at most hospitals as well as in the community at large. There are also certified massage therapists readily available.

Prior to the development of chiropractic as a philosophy of health care, the healing properties of human touch were satisfied by the ancient art of massage. Massage, also called massology, is defined as the systematic manual or mechanical manipulations of the soft tissues of the body by such movements as rubbing, kneading, pressing, rolling, slapping, and tapping for the purpose of promoting circulation of the blood and lymph, relaxation of muscles, relief from pain, restoration of metabolic balance, and other benefits both physical and mental.

The derivation of the word *massage* most likely stems from the Greek word *massage,* which means to knead with the hands. The Arabian word *mass* or *mash* also means to press softly.

Massage is one of the earliest remedial practices of humankind and is said to be the most natural and instinctive means of relieving pain and discomfort. When a person has sore, aching muscles, abdominal pains, or a bruise or wound, it is a natural and instinctive impulse to touch and rub that part of the body to obtain relief. Historical records document that massage was practiced by the Chinese as early as 3000 B.C.

By the 16th century, medical practitioners began to employ massage as part of their healing treatments. Ambroise Pare (1517-1590), a French barber surgeon and one of the founders of modern surgery and inventor of the ligation of arteries, published his theories on massage as an adjunct to the healing process.

However, modern therapy is credited to Dr. Johann Mezger (1839-1909) of Holland, who established the practice and art of massage as a scientific subject for physicians in the remedial treatment of disease.

Today the generally recognized massage schools or philosophies can be divided into the Swedish, Japanese, French, English, and German systems. In addition, minor schools exist around the unique techniques contained in polarity therapy, the Trager method, and reflexology.

There is no doubt that massage has direct psychological and

physiological benefits. Physically, massage increases metabolism, hastens healing, relaxes and refreshes the muscles, and improves the detoxifying functions of the lymphatic system. Massage helps to prevent muscle cramps and spasms, assists the digestive process in assimilation of nutrients, and improves circulation of blood to all body systems. Since blood carries nutrients to the skin, massage is beneficial in keeping the skin functioning in a normal, healthy manner. Psychologically massage relieves fatigue, reduces tension, calms the nervous system, and promotes a sense of relaxation and renewed energy.[6]

Massage reached, perhaps, its most systematic application in traditional Chinese medicine, a system that is one of the subjects of our next chapter.

7

Ancient Medical Traditions:
Chinese/East Indian

The oldest detailed description of traditional Chinese medicine and acupuncture was first documented in the book *Nei Ching* written in approximately 2600 B.C., otherwise known as the *Yellow Emperor's Classic of Internal Medicine*. The translation from Chinese into the English word *acupuncture* came later, from the Greek words *acus* meaning needle and *punctura* meaning puncture. The *Nei Ching*, one of the oldest Chinese medical books in existence, is still used today as one of the main reference books on acupuncture theory.

Since the time of the Yellow Emperor, the practice of acupuncture has remained virtually unchanged. Acupuncture needles dating from 4,000 years ago have been found by archaeologists in China. The first needles were made from stone; later, gold, silver, or bronze was used.

Acupuncture, although one of the mainstays of Oriental medicine, was not introduced into the United States on a large scale until President Richard Nixon's trip to China in 1970. During this diplomatic mission, James Reston, President Nixon's press secretary, became ill and required an appendectomy. What made this surgery noteworthy was the fact that it was performed while Reston was anesthetized with acupuncture as the only method of anesthesia.

Impressed with what had happened, President Nixon encouraged the cultural exchange of medical practitioners between the United States and China. Later that same year, thirty Chinese acupuncturists were invited to participate in a program at the University of California at Los Angeles Medical School. Today, twenty years later, the pain center at UCLA continues to use acupuncture as one of its main modalities for the relief of chronic pain.

Basic acupuncture theory is derived from the ancient philosophy of Taoism. The Taoists believe that the universe can be described by the dualistic concept of yin and yang. All matter is made of yin and yang, including every part of the human body. The concept of yin has been described as that which is dark, cold, moist, yielding, negative in polarity, and feminine. The concept of yang is described as that which is light, warm, dry, dominant, positive in polarity, and masculine.

Although yin and yang have opposite natures, it is their inherent ability to balance each other that creates the dynamic condition that we call health. To the Chinese physician, all diseases or conditions can be classified as either yin or yang in nature due to the imbalance of one to the other. An example of a yin disease would be a chronic, long-standing, degenerative condition, such as cancer. An example of a yang disease would be an acute condition of short duration, such as a flu or sore throat. The Chinese physician manipulates the balance of yin and yang by interacting with the body's energy field using acupuncture points.[1]

According to classical Chinese medicine, the body has approximately 354 energy points, located on the twelve meridians of the body. These twelve meridians or energy loops connect to the six "solid organs" (called yin) — which include the heart, liver, kidney, lung, spleen, and pericardium — and the six "hollow organs" (called yang) — which include the small intestine, gall bladder, bladder, large intestine, stomach, and what is known as the three burners. There are also eight "odd," or extra, meridians that have no direct connection with the twelve main internal organs.

While the exact number of energy points located on the body is a controversial issue currently, classical acupuncture delineated 354 points.[2] Manipulation of the flow of energy throughout the body by utilizing the knowledge of these acupuncture points and meridians is the basis of traditional Chinese health care.

Central to the belief structure of any Chinese physician is the belief in the existence of an energy field, that not only surrounds the human body, but also defines it as being either healthy or diseased. While a Western allopathic physician may describe disease as the clinical manifestation of a particular symptom, a Chinese physician would define disease as an imbalance of energy in a person's physiology.

By energy, they are certainly not referring to anything measurable in terms of musculoskeletal function or caloric intake. The concept of energy is as fundamental to Chinese medicine as ordinary pharmaceuticals are to Western medicine. They define energy by the use of the word *chi.*

Chi refers to the central life force of energy that is the basis of physical existence as we know it. Disease, to a Chinese physician, is nothing more than an imbalance of energy manifested in a particular physiology at a given time. Conversely, health, to a Chinese physician, would be the natural harmony of energy throughout the various meridians of the body.

While a thorough explanation of Chinese medicine and acupuncture is not warranted at this time, a brief description of its assumptions and treatment modalities is in order so that the allopathic physician will better understand the experiences and options open to his/her patient in the alternative health-care system.

Although traditional Chinese medicine is predominantly known by an increasing familiarity with acupuncture in the Western hemisphere, the system itself is much broader in scope and contains acupuncture as only a small part of its therapeutic modalities.

Classical Chinese medicine includes, number one, the four methods of diagnosis:

a) Diagnosis by visual examination

b) Diagnosis by listening to sounds from different parts of the body, as well as examining the characteristics of smells or odors

c) Examination by questioning, especially into any changes in taste

d) Examination by palpation.

Number two, identification and classification of syndromes into eight categories:

a) yin (–) and yang (+)

b) superficial and deep

c) emptiness and fullness

d) coldness and hotness.

Number three, determination of etiology of a disease or symptom from three major categories or causative factors. These three etiological causes can be generalized into:

a) environmental (weather and climate)

b) emotional in origin

c) dietary or activity in origin (including overwork and fatigue).[3]

In prevailing traditional Chinese medical theory, once the patient's syndromes are classified into any of the preceding eight categories or syndromes, methods of treatment will be automatically determined. This is called "treatment based on the classification of syndromes."[4]

As the following charts delineate, based on a particular syndrome, some variable usage of acupuncture and moxibustion (heat stimulus to acupuncture points) treatment will be administered.

8 Categories of Syndromes	Indications and Conditions for Acupuncture and Moxibustion Treatment
1. Yang (+)	Depth of needle must be shallow. Do not let needle stay. Removal of needle must be fast. Apply acupuncture more often, apply less moxibustion.
2. Yin (–)	Depth of needle must be deeper. Removal of needle must be slower. Apply acupuncture more often, apply less moxibustion.
3. Superficial	Depth of needle must be shallow. Apply less moxibustion.
4. Deep	Depth of needle must be deep. Apply more moxibustion.
5. Empty	Method of filling: apply more moxibustion, less acupuncture.
6. Full	Method of discharging: more acupuncture, less moxibustion.
7. Cold	Acupuncture is suitable for deep penetration. Let needle stay. Use more moxibustion.
8. Hot	Acupuncture is suitable fr shallow entry of needle. Can allow bleeding from acupuncture points.

Furthermore, both Yin (–) and Yang (+) are subdivided into 3 levels of intensity: For Yin, – – –, – –, –. For Yang, +++, ++, +. Then the question is, how do you determine these 8 categories of syndromes? In order to identify and classify syndromes into these 8 categories of syndromes, some of the characteristics of emptiness, fullness, coldness, and hotness in 4 methods of diagnosis are shown in the following table (see characteristics of remaining 4 categories of syndromes in the text).   5

More current variations of moxibustion have been recently developed. These include electrical stimulation of a point by sending minute amounts of pulsed current into the needle. These electrical impulses can be adjusted both for frequency and intensity and are typically generated by a small battery-powered device. The Chinese are also experimenting with laser light as a means of stimulating the acupuncture points.

Although the exact mechanism that would explain how acupuncture works is still unknown, recent studies by Dr. Bruce Pomeranz at the University of Toronto have provided insight into how acupuncture affects pain.

				Response to	
			Pressure	Palpation	
Empty			Comfortable	Soft	
Full			Painful	Hard	
	Diagnosis	Appearance	Voice	Symptoms	Pulse
	Syndromes	Viewing	Listening	Questioning	Palpation
MOX. +Ac.	Empty	Pale Complexion, tired and mentally exhausted	Low-pitched voice, light breath	Sweating or night sweating, diarrhea	Weak, forceless weak
AC. +Mox.	Full	Reddish face, euphoria	Disordered speech, with loud voice, heavy, rough breath	Distension of abdomen, constipation, yellowish urine	Strong, forceful
	Cold	Pale blue lips, lies with folded legs	Low-pitched voice	No thirst, cold. limbs, diarrhea	Slow movement
	Hot	Disturbed, worrisome, dry lips, red face	Low and rough heavy-pitched voice, disordered speech	Fever, thirsty, hard feces, yellowish red urine	Fast movement

MOX + Ac.	Moxibustion is the main treatment. supplemented by a little acupuncture	AC. +Mox.	Acupuncture is the main treatment supplemented by a little moxibustion

6

Dr. Pomeranz found that acupuncture was able to stimulate the production of endorphins, opiate-like substances produced in the brain whose function is to control pain in the body. Endorphins have been found to be nearly a thousand times stronger than morphine. Along with the release of endorphins, another substance, called cortisol, is simultaneously released. Coritsol is the body's own natural anti-inflammatory drug. Knowing these facts, it is now clear why acupuncture works so well for joint and structural disorders.[7]

While the complete mechanism of acupuncture's effects on the human body as a whole is not known, it is important to realize that traditional recommendations are based on empiric findings over centuries; and regardless of whether or not one can adequately explain the theory behind the technique, useful information can be gleaned from these historical records.

It is interesting to note from these charts that the Chinese medical practitioner does not determine a disease state by making a diagnosis of a specific organ affected. Rather, they attempt to examine the whole human being and to properly categorize the patient as to a particular syndrome. Western physicians, by contrast, become so specialized in a particular organ system that they may overlook the condition of the rest of the body in formulating their diagnosis and treatment.

In classical Chinese medicine the diagnosis of an ailment begins with the holistic view of the patient as he walks in the door. How the patient looks, how the patient smells, how the patient carries himself, etc., are all essential to the determination of a diagnostic theory.

It is interesting to note that this closely parallels East Indian, or Ayurvedic, medicine as well, where the diagnosis is likewise determined by very concrete, externally observable differences among individuals; such as body habitus, tendency to be hot or cold, sleep patterns, taste preferences, and overall energy level.

Notably, in both traditional Chinese medicine and Indian or Ayurvedic medicine, a primary diagnostic tool is that of pulse diagnosis. While the Western physician takes a single pulse looking for qualities such as rate, rhythm, and strength, both the Chinese and East Indian physician take a pulse that is infinitely more complex and useful to them.

The Chinese practitioner will place three fingers on the radial pulse at the radial styloid of the wrist and determine nine different pulses, each corresponding to a different organ system and each to a different main energy meridian.

If the training and consciousness of the practitioner are sensitive enough, any diagnosis can be derived merely by taking the pulse and correctly identifying the imbalance of energy from one meridian to the next. Once correctly identified, the Chinese practitioner will then use needle acupuncture and/or shiatsu (finger pressure on the acupuncture points themselves) to regulate the energy back to a more evenly balanced homeostasis.

Currently it certainly represents a "stretch" for the allopathic physician to believe that diagnosis and/or treatment based on these energy meridians can detect early cancer or treat it. Only a few years ago the Western medical community was skeptical about acupuncture altogether. Yet, in recent years exhibitions of intracranial surgery as well as open heart surgery have been given worldwide with the use of acupuncture alone as an anesthetic.

The East Indian or Ayurvedic system likewise utilizes pulse diagnosis as one of its main diagnostic modalities. Unlike the Chinese, who base their belief on an energy meridian system, the Ayurvedic physician believes perfect health is a balance of three forces called the "doshas" (vata, pitta, and kapha).

Ayurveda comes from two Sanskrit root words — *ayus*, or life, and *veda*, meaning knowledge or science. Therefore, Ayurveda is usually translated as the science of life. According to Dr. Deepak Chopra, an alternate and more precise reading would be "the knowledge of life span."[8]

The purpose of Ayurveda is to tell us how our lives can be influenced, shaped, extended, and ultimately controlled without interference from sickness or old age. The foundation of Ayurveda is not an exogenous remedy, be it herbal or pharmaceutical. The basis of Ayurveda is the understanding of the mind-body relationship.

When the mind is able to achieve a state of perfect balance, that balance then can be extended to the body. It is this state of balanced awareness, more than any kind of physical immunity, that creates the state of "perfect health" Dr. Chopra alludes to in his book *Perfect Health*:

> "There exists in every person a place that is free
> from disease, that never feels pain, that cannot
> age or die. When you go to this place, limitations
> which all of us accept cease to exist. They are not
> even entertained as a possibility. This is the place
> called perfect health."[9]

Like most of the more naturalistic-based health-care delivery systems, Ayurveda believes your body knows what is good and bad for it; in other words, nature has built the correct instincts into us from birth. The ability to achieve perfect health depends on one's ability to notice and obey these innate tendencies given to us in the inherited intelligence of our physiology.

According to Ayurveda, once we become in tune with our physiology, we are capable of achieving this natural balance (which promotes perfect health) on our own and with a minimal effort on our part.

Fortunately for the practitioner, Ayurveda presents a detailed and comprehensive philosophy, a road map if you will, to make this process easy. The first step in discovering the inherent tendencies of one's physiology is to discover which of the ten basic body types the patient/consumer has.

When an Ayurvedic doctor knows your body type, the theory holds that can then tell which diet, physical activities he, and medical therapies should help an individual patient. Body type also tells the practitioner which activities might do no good or even cause harm. Remembering that the basis of Ayurveda is the mind-body relationship, it would be more accurate to call our body type a "psychophysiological constitutional type." This phrase includes both the mind (psyche) and the body (physiology) in an interdependent state.[10]

The interconnection between the mind and the body is defined in Ayurveda as the doshas. This is that magical place scientists have been searching for where thought turns into matter.

While this may sound quite esoteric, a simple example can explain this point. If a child is afraid of the dark, his fear takes physical shape in the form of adrenaline. The fear itself is clearly mental, yet the adrenaline is clearly physical. Thus, thought has been turned into matter.

The three doshas are defined as vata, pitta, and kapha. Although they regulate thousands of bodily functions, they have three basic functions:

1. vata dosha — controls movement

2. pitta dosha — controls metabolism

3. kapha dosha — controls structure

Although there are only three doshas, Ayurveda combines them in ten possible ways to arrive at ten different body types. Characteristics of the vata type include:

1. light, thin build

2. performs activity quickly

3. irregular hunger and digestion

4. light, interrupted sleep, insomnia

5. enthusiasm, vivaciousness, imagination

6. excitability, changing moods

7. quick to grasp new information, also quick to forget

8. tendency to worry

9. tendency toward constipation

10. tires easily, tendency to overexert

11. mental and physical energy comes in bursts

Characteristics of the pitta type include:

1. medium build

2. medium strength and endurance

3. sharp hunger and thirst, strong digestion

4. tendency toward anger, irritability under stress

5. fair or ruddy skin, often freckled

6. aversion to sun, hot weather

7. enterprising character, likes challenges

8. sharp intellect

9. precise, articulate speech

10. cannot skip meals

11. blond, light brown, or red hair (or reddish undertones)

Characteristics of the kapha type include:

1. solid, powerful build; great physical strength and endurance

2. steady energy; slow and graceful in action

3. tranquil, relaxed personality; slow to anger

4. cool, smooth, thick, pale, often oily skin

5. slow to grasp new information, but good retentive memory

6. heavy, prolonged sleep

7. tendency to obesity

8. slow digestion, mild hunger

9. affectionate, tolerant, forgiving

10. tendency to be possessive, complacent

Most people will find upon reviewing these basic body types that they have characteristics found in all three. This is because body types rarely are of one dosha only. If one dosha is much higher than the other, then one could have a single dosha type. But more commonly, one will have characteristics of either two or three doshas; and thus a possible of ten combinations exists despite only three primary building blocks.[11]

The goal of the Ayurvedic physician and patient is to balance the three doshas. When these doshas are in perfect balance, a state of "perfect health" naturally arises. By balancing the doshas, the Ayurvedic physician does not attempt to achieve equal amounts of vata, pitta, and kapha in any one individual. One's body type is fixed from birth. It does not change.

However, the doshas constantly change. Their nature is to be in constant flux. While one cannot change the ratio of doshas that one was born with, what one can do and must do, according to the Ayurvedic physician, is find the balance that is right for each dosha in each particular patient. By achieving proper balance, one can avoid the various diseases that individual body types are prone to.

Vata types are prone to insomnia, chronic constipation, nervous stomach, anxiety and depression, muscle spasm or cramps, PMS, irritable bowel, chronic pain, high blood pressure, and arthritis.

Pitta types are prone to rashes, acne, heartburn, peptic ulcers, early balding and premature grey hair, poor eyesight, hostility, self-criticism, and heart attacks related to stress.

Kapha types are prone to obesity, congested sinuses, chest colds, painful joints, asthma and/or allergies, depression, diabetes, high cholesterol, and chronic sluggishness in the morning.[12]

According to Ayurveda, the disease process has six distinct phases or steps. The first three are largely invisible and would not be detected by either the physician or the patient. The last three manifest their symptoms and could be detected by both.

The Ayurvedic physician has four broad areas of intervention to attempt to achieve the balance of one's doshas. These four are diet, exercise, daily routine, and seasonal routine.

Like his Chinese counterpart, the Ayurvedic physician relies heavily on the technique of pulse diagnosis. The balance of the doshas can be gleaned from a practitioner who is familiar with proper pulse interpretation.

Similar to acupuncture, ancient Ayurvedic texts locate certain junction points vital to the practitioner for a therapeutic intervention. These points are called "marmas," of which there are 107. Although they are invisible to the eye, these marmas are accessible through the sense of touch and are considered critical for maintaining balance throughout the body.

It is interesting to note the extreme similarity between these points and the Chinese acupuncture meridian system. Historically, Ayurvedic marma therapy predates the Chinese approach, and it is likely that acupuncture was a development of it.

Perhaps the most startling and controversial belief of the Ayurvedic system is the concept that aging is neither necessary nor correct. As Deepak Chopra states, "Although everyone falls prey to the aging process, no one has ever proved that it is necessary."[13]

According to the ancient sages of Ayurveda, who have been renowned for their own advanced longevity, aging is no more than a "mistake of the intellect." This mistake consists of identifying oneself solely with the physical body in its limited state defined in time and space. The cure for this is to correct the intellect's mistake and identify oneself with the quantum mechanical body instead.

In other words, it is Ayurvedic medicine's belief that by contacting the quantum ground state of the mind through the process of meditation, the properties this ground state contains will naturally and spontaneously express themselves in the functioning physiology of the body. Since the mind and body are intimately connected, it does make sense that habitual contact of a specific quality by use of the attention will produce a corresponding physiological correlate.

Nonetheless, to insist that aging is unnecessary is quite a philosophical jump. It is not within the scope of this text to debate this issue here.

It is however, interesting to observe that studies conducted on practitioners of the Transcendental Meditation technique have shown that with continued practice of meditation, one's chronological age and one's biological age need not follow the same pattern as the nonmeditating cohort group.

These original studies, performed by Dr. Keith Wallace, used three measures that change uniformly in the general population as people age: near-point vision, acuity of hearing, and systolic blood pressure.

Since all three of these are known to deteriorate steadily over time, they give a reliable approximation of the biological age of the whole body at a given chronological age. Dr. Wallace found that meditation made his subjects biologically younger than their years would indicate — and by a considerable amount. These studies have subsequently been repeated and confirmed elsewhere.[14]

It is worth noting that the two oldest systems of medicine both believe in some type of natural balance of energy forces as a sign of health. The fact that they have slightly different names and are manipulated differently does not detract from their overall similarity and holistic viewpoint of health as a natural physiologic state to be aspired to.

Both the traditional Chinese system and the traditional East Indian system have multiple offshoots in treatment and diagnostic forms, which originate from this basic concept. I shall mention just a few of the more common Chinese practices here in passing.

T'ai chi, with which I have much personal experience, is a regimen of systemized movements believed to promote health in its practitioner. These movements are done very slowly and gracefully and compose not only part of ancient Chinese dance and martial art, but are also a source of personal care to promote optimum health.

It is the belief that various movements promote the release or transference of energy from one part of the body to another, creating a systematic and repeatable state of harmonious functioning in the individual. Advanced practitioners of t'ai chi have been known to demonstrate enormous vitality and strength even in advanced years.

In countries such as China, which I had the good fortune to visit in 1989 on a medical mission, it is inspiring to watch the entire population performing t'ai chi outside at five o'clock in the morning. One of the highlights of my life was receiving an ovation from a number of onlookers while I performed t'ai chi with the local populous in the early morning hours.

While t'ai chi is an exercise designed to promote good health in general, chi gong is the medical application of specific movements to achieve precise desired results. Significant basic research is currently being conducted by the Chinese government as to the efficacy of chi gong in treating such diseases as cancer.

By the practice of chi gong, the manipulation of energy fields over experimental conditions can be controlled and measured. One such experiment altered the rate of malignant cell mutation within cells growing in a petri dish. Other experiments have altered the life span of diseased laboratory animals.[15] Masters of chi gong are becoming increasingly more available in our country and are readily treating and teaching people this technique as a means of personal health preservation.

The "pop culture" of alternative health-care options also includes more esoteric modalities relating to energy balancing techniques, such as color and aromatherapy techniques. It is the belief of all of these types of practitioners and consumers that they, too, can in some way affect the consumer's energy field in such a way that is repeatable and verifiable, thus promoting health.

As esoteric and foreign to the allopathic physician as these concepts may seem, one can scarcely argue with their ability to withstand the test of time and promote health in their individual cultures.

> "I once heard a rumor about an Indian sage who remarked at his surprise that Americans would trust their psychic health to the unproven discipline of psychiatry. "After all," he explained, the science of psychiatry is less than one hundred years old, and meditation is five thousand years old."

It was his belief that in the future, meditation will be found scientifically to be the cure of most psychiatric problems.

8

The Mind-Body Connection

It should come as no surprise to the modern allopathic physician that the mind-body connection plays a central role in both the disease and the health process. All of psychiatry as well as psychology are fundamentally based on this assumption. There is no better demonstration of the intimate relationship between psychological state and physiology than the case studies cited in Michael Talbot's book *The Holographic Universe*. According to Talbot, the clinical data of multiple-personality disorders is incontrovertible evidence that illness is largely a drama of the psyche played out in biology.

He cites the case of an acute medical condition possessed by one personality, which suddenly vanishes when another personality takes over within the same physical body. For example, all but one of the multiple selves of a man were acutely allergic to orange juice, breaking out in a rash after consumption. But if the "host" switched to his nonallergic subpersonality, the rash instantly disappeared, and he could drink orange juice with no negative reaction.

Another case cited by Talbot describes a patient whose eye was stung by a wasp, causing it to swell shut. He was in such great pain that his psychiatrist induced a change in personality to a new self that had not been stung by the wasp. Remarkably, the man's pain and swelling disappeared. Evidence such as this brings Michael Talbot to the conclusion that: "The body is a hologram of consciousness and mentally distributed throughout the system. . . . Our body listens to everything we think and feel. It takes our wishes literally, so we must be vigilant."[1]

But the concept of the mind-body connection as it exists in Western medicine is an infant compared to the significance it achieves in ancient traditional systems (Chinese and East Indian).

In these traditional medical practices, the existence of an energy field around the body and within the body is not merely that of a structural phenomenon but, more important, that of a primal phenomenon. The primacy of this conception is best illustrated by the beliefs and usage of techniques of meditation.

Various forms of meditation inducing altered states of consciousness have probably existed since the beginning of man's appearance on earth. They can be found in all primitive cultures as well as all major religions. Types of meditation readily available include meditation techniques based on visualization, concentration, chanting, mantra, kundilini, and tantric among others.

Regardless of the type of meditation practiced, a belief that meditation can contact and alter the primal force of life in some predictable way is common to all these various traditions.

For the more ancient healing systems (Chinese and East Indian), human consciousness represents the source, course, and dominant reality of this energy field that is to be diagnosed and manipulated. It would not be incorrect to say that for these practitioners and consumers, consciousness itself is imbued with an almost infinite potential and power.

The idea that human consciousness exists as the fundamental building block of creation and even as the ground state of quantum mechanics is not an idea that is new to current philosophy, physics, or medicine.[2] Dr. Deepak Chopra, who has been the best-selling author of alternative medical books for the past five years, clearly describes the primacy of consciousness as central to his medical philosophy.

Detailed discussion of this concept is clearly beyond the scope of this book. But suffice it to say that many practitioners of meditation believe that by contacting the source of consciousness, they contact "a field of all possibilities" and "a field of infinite correlation" from which they can promote the evolution of their central nervous system and achieve the goal of perfect health.

Whether meditation, visualization, and even "faith healing" truly exist on a quantum mechanical level and contain inherent within them this type of potentiality is something that only the future will be able to tell scientifically. This type of data is already being reviewed by such authors as Daniel J. Benor. In his original article "Complimentary Medical Research," published in 1990, he reviewed 131 controlled trials that look at the variable of the mind's influence on the healing process. These experiments deal with healing effects on enzymes, cells, yeasts, bacteria, plants, animals, and human beings.[3]

Similarly, the issue of prayer and its relationship to medicine is dealt with very nicely in Dr. Dossey's book *Healing Words*. It may surprise the allopathic medical student to know that experiments with people have showed that prayer positively affects high blood pressure, wounds, heart attacks, headaches, and anxiety. Subjects in these studies have also included the manipulation of water, enzymes, bacteria, fungi, yeast, red blood cells, cancer cells, pacemaker cells, seeds, plants, algae, moth larvae, mice, and chicks.

Among the processes that have been variables in these studies are activity of enzymes, the growth rates of leukemic white blood cells, mutation rates of bacteria, germination and growth rates of various seeds, the firing rate of pacemaker cells, healing rates of wounds, the size of goiters and tumors, the time required to awaken from anesthesia, autonomic effects such as electrodermal activity of the skin, rates of hemolysis of red blood cells, and hemoglobin levels.[4]

While the existence of the aforementioned studies investigating prayer may surprise the medical community, research on meditation has been commonplace. Repeated scientific experiments have demonstrated that very concrete benefits to overall health are gained from the regular practice of meditation. Hundreds of studies have documented positive results with diverse variables ranging from decreasing oxygen consumption and lactic acid production to more esoteric-sounding results, such as a decreased crime rate in a given locality when one percent of the surrounding population practices meditation.[5]

The basic assumption underlying meditation's less esoteric claims is that *rest is the basis of activity.* Commonsensically, the greater one's level of rest, the more dynamic, creative, and efficient the level of activity will be — one can view meditation as the ultimate form of stress management.

Eastern meditation often uses the analogy between meditation and activity as that of drawing an arrow back on a bow. The farther we draw back the arrow, the greater its potential and higher degree of accuracy. When we finally let go of the arrow from this dormant and latent state of being pulled back, it springs into activity with fresh dynamism.[6]

The basic mechanism proposed for the beneficial effect of meditation is that three things occur during the process:

1. The meditative practitioner achieves a state of metabolic rest deeper than deep sleep; spontaneously the body undergoes a purification of "stress" that is ordinarily not relieved during sleep or dream state;

2. Accompanying this decrease of metabolic rate (deeper than sleep) is the expansion of consciousness rather than the dissolution of consciousness or awareness as we know it defining deep sleep;

3. The process of meditation, by repeatedly decreasing the metabolic rate, is in and of itself a mechanism for decreasing the energy expenditure of the body.

It is interesting to note how central the concept of energy conservation and harmony is to all of the more Eastern health-care philosophies. One can look at the conservation of energy as a common denominator running through the practices of meditation, fasting, and even the belief that maintaining silence (i.e., not speaking) promotes natural healing of the body's physiology.

As a practitioner of meditation for over twenty years who has also dabbled experimentally in both fasting and the maintenance of silence, I can attest to the tremendous energy one is able to gain by limiting the outward flow of attention and action from the body.

I find it notable that even in our Western tradition, the Greek philosopher Plato alluded to a turning inward of all energies and attention in order to gain great knowledge. Plato referred to his technique of meditation as "the dialectic." He mentions the process of meditating throughout *The Republic* as "practicing death." By this he means to accustom the soul to "withdraw from all contact with the body and concentrate itself by itself . . . alone by itself."[7]

9

A New Paradigm/Model of Health-Care Delivery

It would be wrong of me to merely list the availability of each of these systems and their rationales without attempting to synthesize all of this information into a useful format. Having been a physician for almost fifteen years, I have spent much of my time and energy attempting to make sense of the myriad of health-care systems presented in this book.

Science is an ongoing process. We build a model or paradigm, which is no more than an attempt to explain the phenomena that we experience in the external world. It is only the predictive value of any given model that makes it useful. In other words, if a model or paradigm ceases to be able to predict an outcome to a high statistical degree of probability, then it no longer is a useful model and should be discarded.

It is my belief that the allopathic system of Western medical education viewed in isolation represents an endangered model. Any physician who is sensitive and truthful with himself/herself continues to agonize over his/her inability to provide the patient with a higher degree of medical success.

How many times have each of us, either as a physician or as a health-care consumer, treated one ailment only to see another pop up in its place? Perhaps, as the more ancient health sciences allude to, a truly holistic view of the body and mind must be understood in order to achieve a true balance in physiology that promotes optimum health.

I have absolutely no personal interest in "bashing" the allopathic Western medical profession as it now exists. For selected disease processes, injuries, or medical crises it represents one of the finest culminations of applied intelligence that civilization has ever record-ed. However, the fallibility of Western allopathic medicine, from my perspective, is not related to its treatment failures inasmuch as its inability to understand the nature of its own inadequacies and admit its limitations.

For diseases of known genetic mechanisms, advanced structural disintegrations/degenerations, life-threatening crises, or severe trauma (such as a fracture), Western allopathic medicine is extremely effective. Unfortunately these comprise only a small percentage of the total num-ber of disease processes known to man. It is, rather, our inability to embrace systems with a broader viewpoint able to encompass and understand the nature of health itself that may lead to the demise of allopathy. Western medical technology is basically a knee-jerk reflex in response to disease.

The more ancient traditional medical systems are the opposite. They are truly systems of health maintenance that aim at promoting the prevention of disease at an earlier stage by encouraging the practitioner to obtain a state of heightened awareness toward his/her physiology and pursue the goal of perfect health.

It is this lack of an overall unifying concept of health that is at the very heart of allopathic Western medicine's inability to progress. Given the fact that these very detailed, complex, and in some sense time-proven systems already exist, it behooves Western medical science to deeply investigate them through the gift of advanced scientific research in order to document the parts that are efficacious and the parts that are not.

An Indian sage once said that the steps of progress are as fol-
lows: stability, adaptability, integration, purification, and
growth.[1]

This seemingly simple statement contains a great deal of useful
information regarding any evolutionary process. One has to be "stable"
in order to have the foundation to withstand change. We have that stability now in the wealth of information each of our medical systems
contains. Yet one has to be "adaptable" in order to synthesize the best of
each of these systems and discard the ineffective aspects time has taught
us are unnecessary.

The ability to sort through the good and bad of any system is the
process of "integration." Once we synthesize a new master system from
all of the previously existing medical systems to date, we will have
achieved the process of integration.

The next step of "purification" then ensues. Time will tell us which
of our changes have been most effective and which should continue to
remain in this master system. This is the process of purification. The
system will spontaneously purify previous adjustments that have been
found lacking and are no longer necessary. As this entire process continues to take place, the health-care system as we know it should continue
to grow and evolve.

It is my belief that these very processes need to occur in order to
move forward with the development of a true health-care system.

The wonderful thing about free-market enterprise is that the market undergoes spontaneous shifts and corrections. An example is the
downsizing of American companies over the past ten to fifteen years as a
more global economy/market has developed.

The same is true of health care. It exists within the free enterprise
system, and the market correction has already taken place.[2] It is now
time, however, to downsize our Western medical system and realign our
product with consumer/patient demands and expectations.

It is difficult to imagine what form this actually will take in the
United States. I find it hard to picture the entrenched bureaucracy of
Western medical schools accepting the more esoteric and "scientifically
unproven" philosophies of the alternative health-care industry. Perhaps
the only solution possible will resemble the health-care delivery system
of China.

In China two health-care systems exist side by side. The patient/consumer can choose to enter building "A", which houses traditional Chinese medical-care practitioners (acupuncture/herbal medicine), or building "B," which houses a more primitive form of Western allopathic medicine than we have in this country.

Imagine the greater power a synthesis of the old and new health-care systems potentially could offer.

I propose the following synthesis as a basis to begin:

1. The primacy of "health" is a recognizable goal as opposed to the knee-jerk reaction of treating disease as it arises.

2. This personal goal of "perfect health" exists as the primary responsibility of the patient as opposed to the responsibility of the health-care professional.

3. The development of perfect health is truly a lifelong endeavor by the patient and should form the basis for much of his/her style of living.

   An example would be the avoidance of all influences known to be deleterious to a healthy, functioning physiology (tobacco, excessive food, alcohol, or drug usage) and to embrace all those influences that promote a balanced physiology (proper rest, diet, exercise).

4. Given the basic assumption that rest is the basis of activity and the better the quality of the rest the more dynamic the quality of one's activity, I would recommend some form of meditation to all individuals.

Certainly there exist hundreds of techniques of meditation, and each individual may be more or less attracted to various techniques than others. It is my personal bias, based on the experience of having tried many other forms of meditation as well as being a certified teacher of meditation and t'ai chi, that most people adapt best to a mantra-type meditation (such as Transcendental Meditation [TM] as taught by Maharishi Mahesh Yogi). I recommend it both for its uniformity in teaching, exactly the same worldwide, and its adaptability to all lifestyles.

Unique to the Transcendental Meditation program is the fact that no belief in the technique itself is required nor is any alteration of lifestyle or religion necessary.[3] One merely adopts to one's already established routine a twenty-minute practice twice daily.[4]

The basic assumption is that by exposing one's nervous system to a quality of rest twice as deep as deep sleep,[5] the regular stress and strain of one's life, which theoretically promotes if not aggravates most of the Western industrialized type disease, would be eradicated.

An analogy for understanding meditation is to consider our nervous system as a twisted rope knotted up with stress. As we continue to contact a field of deeper and deeper rest, the stress begins slowly to unwind and the rope untangles.

There is the inherent assumption that rest alone purifies stress. This is not terribly farfetched when one considers the beneficial qualities of sleep. Ordinary sleep, due to nothing more than the decrease of metabolic rate, allows the body to spontaneously purify some form of biochemical stress. This accumulated stress would actually be life threatening were sleep to be interrupted totally for a number of weeks.

Is it really such a leap of faith to then say that rest many times deeper than sleep should purify a level of stress and strain that the ordinary sleep state does not? This is the basic mechanism behind the belief that regular meditation is an evolutionary technique for the body on a physiological level. There are certainly other more esoteric explanations for meditation's profound effects (the habitual contact with an absolute field of existence beyond time and space, which is in itself a field of infinite possibilities, infinite correlation, perfect intelligence, and full potentiality). But the more esoteric explanations need not fall within the scope of this treatise, as they already exist within current best-sellers elsewhere.[6]

Finally, another common analogy to describe the primacy of meditation in any health-field endeavor must be offered:

> A wise man once commented to his students, "Why paint the leaves of the tree green in order to make it look healthy? This is a superficial and immaterial action. What is necessary to do is water the root of the tree in order to promote its life force and future health."

The message here, of course, is that of interacting with a system at its foundation. In much the same way one would never attend to a diseased tree by painting its leaves green in order to make it look shiny, one should not attempt to interface with the human physiology by treating it piecemeal, symptom by symptom.

A more profound understanding of the holistic view of one's physiology will demonstrate a more all-encompassing mechanism of treatment. Furthermore, as we have already discussed, the need to intervene on the subtlest level possible, because it contains the greatest potential energy to change the future physiology of the patient, is also of primary importance.

Consider the analogy that punching an opponent with a fist is much less deadly than exploding an atom bomb. This illustrates the basic point that nature is organized in a multilevel fashion and that the subtler, more fundamental levels (e.g., nuclear) contain the greatest power and organizing ability. By organizing ability, I mean that intervention at the subtlest possible level will spontaneousxly affect all of the grosser levels. Again, watering the root of the plant spontaneously improves the outward manifestation of its beauty.

Learning from this analogy, it should be obvious that the goal of our newly synthesized health-care system is to interface each disease at the earliest possible (i.e., most subtle) level when appropriate. If we were to rank the various health-care systems from gross to subtle, the following continuum would be seen:

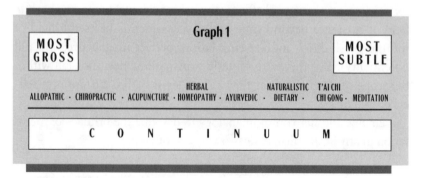

Another equally important continuum that parallels the illustration of the first one is the continuum between doctor-oriented responsibility versus patient-oriented responsibility. If we were to analyze the continuum from gross (allopathic medicine) to subtle (meditation), we find that as we go down the continuum toward meditation, the responsibility of the doctor as the primary care giver diminishes and the responsibility of the patient as his/her own care giver increases.

For example, the traditional allopathic-oriented patient presents himself/herself to his/her physician usually not aware of his/her diagnosis and looking for outside, exogenous intervention to cure his/her symptomatology. Most traditional patients historically fail to even question the doctor regarding their health care, preferring to place their total trust in the physician's care. Furthermore, these types of patients frequently prefer a "quick and easy" solution to any disease state (such as taking an oral medication or an injection or having surgery) as opposed to altering their lifestyle or adopting any type of dramatic change in their behavioral patterns.

By contrast, the patient utilizing meditation is exactly the opposite. It is the patient himself/herself who is in tune with the body and who realigns it with the laws of nature through a self-directed technique.

This continuum of various practices can also be analyzed in terms of the overall treatment scope. Again, the overspecialization of allopathic physicians has led to a piecemeal understanding and an orientation toward disease.

Chiropractic certainly extends a more holistic view to the patient. But depending on the practitioner, this still stays at the very gross level of structural physiology.

Acupuncture becomes more subtle in that it deals with an underlying energy system as opposed to a structural system. But again, this is completely exogenous, as the doctor places the needles in the patient's body and formulates both the diagnosis and treatment. It is certainly not something that patients do to themselves.

Acupuncture, likewise, is a form of manipulation that is physician directed. Being more subtle in its interactive level, the effectiveness of acupuncture takes place through multiple treatment sessions and is not achieved through a single intervention (such as surgery in the allopathic state).

As we progress to t'ai chi/chi gong, we see that the patient assumes responsibility for practicing this exercise on a regular basis, believing it will achieve a natural homeostasis of the body, promoting perfect health.

Nutrition/herbal supplements are similar in that the patient by a change in lifestyle can adopt a very fundamental health-oriented behavior. Although, in the scope of herbal supplements, a health-care professional's advice is usually sought.

The same continuum can be analyzed in terms of crisis orientation versus prevention. Certainly the hallmark of successful allopathic medicine, and where it usually has the greatest value, is in its ability to intervene in a crisis to save a patient's life. Its weakness is in the field of preventative medicine, as it does not have a philosophy or concept of perfect health defined. If one cannot define perfect health, the mechanisms of attaining it obviously are limited.

This continuum can also be analyzed by using our analogy of gross intervention as opposed to subtle intervention. Once again allopathic medicine attempts to interface on the grossest possible level, such as with surgery or powerful drug therapies, which due to their "unnaturalness" may produce extreme side effects.

Chiropractic, because of its primary usage of structural manipulation, also tends to be a grosser interaction with the patient even if it assumes philosophically that one is affecting more subtle energy forces. My skepticism of chiropractic as a primary modality has always been that, like allopathic medicine, structural realignment or manipulation is a very gross form of intervention. And if more subtle changes in the body are not dealt with in a primary fashion, the adjustment/manipulation that the patient has just undergone typically disappears.

My experience has been that many chiropractic patients feel absolutely wonderful when they leave the chiropractor's office only to have the adjustment or manipulation "slip" and then return to their pretreatment symptomatology.

It is more helpful to understand this if one uses the analogy of dyeing cloth to make it colorfast:

> Eastern meditation has been described by using the analogy of
> a white cloth dipping in red dye. We take the white cloth and
> dip it in the red dye over and over until the stain becomes fast.
> Until it no longer can be bleached by the sun. Once this is
> complete, the dye will never fade again.

We see that these natural techniques are a slower and more gradual process. They involve *habituating the nervous system* to a particular experience until the adaptability of the nervous system to accept this experience becomes a constant. A commonsense example is that of the athlete working out in the gym. No one expects to sculpt one's body in a single session. Through the repeated habituation of various exercises, each isolating muscle groups, the muscle tone of the body can be sculpted.

The same is true of cardiac rehabilitation. Repeated anaerobic or aerobic sessions are necessary to build up a state of cardiac health. Why, then, should it be difficult to understand that either through some form of energy manipulation and/or meditation, a gradual habituation of the nervous system to a new beneficial experience will promote a lasting positive effect over time?

Graph 2

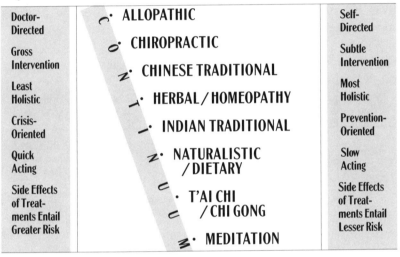

Doctor-Directed	ALLOPATHIC	Self-Directed
Gross Intervention	CHIROPRACTIC	Subtle Intervention
Least Holistic	CHINESE TRADITIONAL	Most Holistic
Crisis-Oriented	HERBAL / HOMEOPATHY	Prevention-Oriented
Quick Acting	INDIAN TRADITIONAL	Slow Acting
Side Effects of Treatments Entail Greater Risk	NATURALISTIC / DIETARY T'AI CHI / CHI GONG MEDITATION	Side Effects of Treatments Entail Lesser Risk

It is important to reiterate at this point that this book makes no attempt to validate any particular system, but rather to present it to the medical student so that he/she has a better comprehension of the various forces active in the current marketplace of health care. It is not my intention to be involved in black-and-white thinking.

I certainly do not claim that any one of these health-care systems is intrinsically wrong or right. Rather, the impression I hope to give is that each particular system may be either better or more poorly suited to interface with a specific disease process at a particular time.

For instance, the strength of allopathic medicine is its ability to deal with diseases of known mechanisms of action or end-stage disease. By known mechanisms of action, we mean disease where a genetic basis is understood or a missing enzyme has been isolated or through the manipulation of a hormone, a more natural homeostasis can be achieved. Perfect examples are phenylketonuria, thyroid disease, or cardiac arrest. We certainly would not begin to treat cardiac arrest by sitting down in meditation or taking herbal medicines. The effects of these techniques would be too slow to avert the disaster.

However, since it has been estimated that more than 50% of all medical care is dealing with symptomatology of psychosomatic origin or stress-induced origin, a more generalized technique such as meditation may be better equipped to prevent the continuing disease process from evolving.

The following graph illustrates the strength and weakness of each particular health-care system in relationship to (1) their model of action, (2) their technique of diagnosis, and (3) their primary mode of treatment:

Graph 3   Gross...   Continuum...

SYSTEM TYPE	ALLOPATHIC	CHIROPRACTIC	TRADITIONAL CHINESE MEDICINE
MODEL	Discover scientific mechanism of disease Genetic /infectious Toxic /inflammatory Neoplastic, etc.	Abnormality of skeletal structure: Blocks proper functioning of physiology (on more subtle levels)	Disease equals an imbalance of energy among organ systems or meridians Dynamic balance between opposing forces of yin and yang
DIAGNOSIS	Least holistic in view Predominance of "laboratory" tests over physical diagnosis	Highly variable by practitioner May include variables of each alternative medical system	Full diagnosis Holistic view of symptoms and presentation
TREATMENT	Most doctor-oriented Least preventative Quicker results Crisis-oriented Least holistic	May include variables of each alternative medical system Unique use of manipulation, which varies by school of origin	Herbal Dietary Exercise Acupuncture (physician-directed) T'ai chi / chi gong (self-directed)

One can see that analysis of this graph provides concepts of intervention that are foreign to us in our present state of medical knowledge. For instance, the traditional allopathic physician may think of a routine stress test as a means of diagnosing heart disease at a preclinical level. Certainly the cardiologist who finds significant changes on a patient's stress test can intervene and change the patient's lifestyle prior to the development of catastrophic cardiac symptoms.

While this certainly may be a fortuitous diagnostic test, it would be erroneous to think that it interfaces with the patient's life in an early/preventative state. Instead, it actually diagnoses a patient's rather severe state of disease on the continuum of cardiac health just prior to its clinical manifestation.

Graph 4   Continuum . . .   Subtle . . .

SYSTEM TYPE	TRADITIONAL INDIAN MEDICINE (AYURVEDA)	HERBAL MEDICINES NATUROPATHY DIET	MEDITATION
MODEL	Disease results from imbalance of three primary forces: Vata / Pitta / Kapha	Disease results from improper lifestyle leading to auto-intoxication	Disease results from nonalliance with the "Laws of Nature" creating stress, causing disease Nonstress state is normalcy or perfect health
DIAGNOSIS	Pulse diagnosis (self-or physician-directed) Holistic view of symptoms and presentation	Holistic view of symptomatology Self-directed or physician-directed Subtle lab test (e.g., hair analysis)	Self-directed based on subjective experience for individual symptom manifestation
TREATMENT	Self-or physician-directed: Dietary · Herbal Exercise (e.g., yoga) Meditation	Preventative Self-directed or physician-directed Herbal· Dietary·Exercise	Preventative by spontaneously aligning one's physiology with the "Laws of Nature" and releasing stress Totally self-directed

Hypothetically, true prevention might have been achieved through proper diet, exercise, and techniques of stress reduction. This is a perfect example of the expanded type of thinking that must take place in order to reap the benefits of a synthesized medical model.

10

The Present Challenge

The true challenge to our health-care system is whether this readily available knowledge will be properly embraced by the existing medical regime. Obviously, the radicalization of health care such as I have proposed is a very threatening concept to the status quo. All established systems are resistant to change, and this resistance is no less manifested in a business than it is in an organism. That is why the evolutionary process is a slow, gradual event occurring over time.

Nonetheless, the reality is that this evolutionary process is already taking place in the marketplace. And if traditional allopathic medicine hopes to continue controlling a dominant market share, it must make room for the realities of an alternative health-care system.

To stick our heads in the sand and refuse to deal with the revolution in health care that is already taking place is for allopathy to sign a death warrant for utilization by a large part of the American public. It is my hope that rather than exclude this segment of the consumer population, orthodox Western medicine will expand its horizons to provide a better product.

The better product, such as a synthesis of the strengths and benefits of the various systems as I have proposed, would allow the orthodox Western medical system to recapture a very large segment of the population now seeking alternative health-care treatments. It would also reestablish the respect that is eroding toward allopathic medical doctors.

As one who was traditionally educated in allopathic medicine, I can attest to the surprise and delight of most patients to various treatment options I give them with a more natural basis.

Traditional allopathic physicians will find much less resistance to these type of changes in their patient/consumer population than in their own medical profession. The historic legal battles between chiropractic and allopathic medicine are perfect examples of the danger of black-and-white thinking producing in-group/out-group strategies.

The next challenge for organizations such as the NIH will be to coordinate research into the efficacy of treatment for each of these respective disciplines. For instance, at the first sign of early hypertension, which system best interfaces with the disease process? Should allopathic pharmaceuticals be used immediately to symptomatically treat the rise in blood pressure, or should the opposite end of the continuum be considered? Should meditation be the first line of treatment to decrease one's blood pressure in lieu of pharmaceuticals? Or perhaps the middle of the continuum provides the best option? Would acupuncture or herbal medicine be a better choice for early hypertension?

Obviously, each alternative health-care system has its own typical risk/benefit ratio. In general, the risks of side effects will be less as we proceed along the continuum toward meditation. But the benefits may evolve more slowly. Thus, the immediacy of a desired result will in most cases dictate the appropriate choice of health-care system.

Finally, in the 1990s no discussion of health-care would be complete without addressing the issue of cost-effectiveness. As our country struggles to revamp the health-care system, the issue of cost-effectiveness becomes critical.

The current debate rages over the proper format by which allopathic medicine should be delivered. Many elaborate arguments are used to analyze the cost-effectiveness of one political solution to another. I would assert that these are tantamount to painting the leaves on a tree and that all solutions will be found wanting.

This is not because doctors are greedy people or are out to cheat the system. Rather, it is because the system itself is fundamentally flawed.

Given the expansive view provided in this book, I hope it is obvious that true cost containment is a much more complex issue than the concept of managed care versus fee-for-service or a single-payer system.

I am certainly not so naive as to think this will be an easy transition. The seeds of resistance to a change of this magnitude exist on many levels. There will be enormous political opposition to open up the venue of health care to what have been heretofore considered "out" groups or "fringe" groups.

There will be, as there already is, an enormous resistance of the FDA to accept the further unregulated arena of health-care products. The pharmaceutical industry, which has enjoyed a virtual monopoly in health care, will certainly be up in arms. The growing resentment and the attempt to control the already burgeoning health-food industry are current political issues. Despite the fact that a 1990 report by the federal government's General Accounting Office (GAO) claims that "51.5% of drugs approved by the FDA have serious postapproval risks including heart failure, birth defects, kidney failure, blindness, and convulsions,"[1] no one seems to be controlling the alliance between the FDA and the pharmaceutical industry. Why is this?

> "The Task Force (FDA) considered many issues in its deliberations including to ensure that the existence of dietary supplements (vitamins, minerals, amino acids, herbs, and other) on the market does not act as a disincentive for drug development." (FDA Task Force Report released June 15, 1993.)[2]

Obviously the federal government and the pharmaceutical industry have a different agenda than the consumer. Why would the federal government want to protect an industry with, according to the GAO report in 1990, profit margins over the past decade that are triple the rate of inflation and of the average Fortune 500 company?[3]

Commenting on the health-care system of his era, an angry young German Swiss doctor said, "The physician's duty is to heal the sick, not to enrich the apothecary." His name was Paracelsus. Historical records from the seventeenth century document that the usual apothecary markup was 300%.[4] With profit motives like these, it is no wonder that some historical commentators believe that "profit has always been more a decisive factor than human misery in medical issues."[5]

Are we doomed to have history repeat itself? If we do not learn from it, we most certainly will. How commonplace is the current saying, "The cure is worse than the disease"?

In the seventeenth century, when almost all standard professional treatments for illness at best were unpleasant and at worst meant total agony, a more natural system of self-care based on folklore developed. As doctoring at this time had an appallingly bad reputation, saving a friend from falling into the clutches of the medical profession by passing on some tried and trusted family recipe for a disorder was rendering a service indeed. This same feeling exists today among patients who utilize alternative heath-care systems.

Are these perceptions exaggerated or unfounded? A review of the following quotations illustrates how widespread and mainstream this has become:

> *"We don't know what we're doing in medicine. . . .*
> *Perhaps one-quarter to one-third of medical services*
> *may be of little or no benefit to patients."*
>
> DR. DAVID EDDY, DIRECTOR,
> DUKE UNIVERSITY HEALTH POLICY RESEARCH[6]

> *"If you're feeling well, just stay away from the doctor."*
>
> EUGENE ROBBINS, M.D., PROFESSOR
> EMERITUS, STANFORD UNIVERSITY[7]

> *"The health-care system is in crisis, if not chaos. If*
> *you really want to beat the system, don't use it."*
>
> C. EVERETT KOOP, M.D.,
> FORMER U.S. SURGEON GENERAL [8]

One can easily see that our fate is precariously balanced. Perhaps, no one has better echoed the present danger we now face than Dr. Benjamin Rush (signer of the Declaration of Independence):

"Unless we put medical freedom into the Constitution, the time will come when medicine will organize itself into an undercover dictatorship. To restrict the art of healing to doctors and deny equal privileges to others will constitute the Bastille of medical science. All such laws are un-American and despotic."[9]

How timely are these words uttered so long ago.

Nor will the vested interests of industry and government be the only sources of resistance. Various religious groups will no doubt object to some forms of meditation as being "Satanic." Nonetheless, I encourage everyone to be brave and forge ahead with true vision toward the goal. And if the goal is to achieve a system designed to promote perfect health and not a system to protect our individual vested interests, the task should not be impossible to achieve.

Perhaps the true and more valid stumbling block to swift achievement of this project is that our scientific method has its limits. As powerful as twentieth-century science has become, the ability to document subtle changes, such as those presented in this book, are very difficult to quantitate. For example, in order to truly assess the cost-effectiveness of various alternative health-care systems compared to allopathic medicine, many years, if not decades, will be required to collect data.

Enormous political pressure must be brought to bear before change will take place. No bureaucracy will willingly decrease its control over a segment of the population or its budget. Yet since the evolution of health care as I have illustrated it calls for reempowerment of the consumer and a lesser control by the current establishment, this must inevitably be the case. Is it still possible to turn back the hands of time and achieve that correct mixture of technological advancement and individual simplicity that Ivan Illich dreams about?

"A world of optimal and widespread health is obviously a world of minimal and only occasional medical intervention. Healthy people are those who live in healthy homes on a healthy diet in an environment equally fit for birth, growth, work, healing, and dying; they are sustained by a culture that enhances the conscious acceptance of limits to population, of aging, of incomplete recovery and ever imminent death. Healthy people need minimal bureaucratic interference to mate, give birth, share the human condition, and die."[10]

11

In Conclusion

In conclusion, let me sympathize with you, the consumer, for the horrible mess our health-care system is in and with you, the medical students, in your present plight. It was not that many years ago that as a young medical student I was asked to imbibe a body of knowledge overwhelming in its breadth as well as depth. It is, perhaps, an impossible achievement to be current with the generalized scope of medical knowledge as it now exists.

I am certainly aware of the burden this challenge places upon the beginning medical student at this time. The last thing one wishes to confront is an entire new body of knowledge, let alone an entire new philosophy of thinking, while starting one's new career.

The fact that this is controversial in nature is even more upsetting to the student at this level. It is hard enough to progress and succeed with medical education as it is currently designed without rocking the boat. I know firsthand the profound identity crisis that can result from trying to incorporate such seemingly diametrically opposed bodies of knowledge. One is confronted with the issue of one's basic philosophy in becoming a physician altogether.

This is, of course, a very difficult thing to do when one is at such an early stage in medical training. I did not feel comfortable presenting this information in a public venue until thirteen years after my medical-school graduation. Once one is already an established practitioner both in technique and in business, it is much easier to adapt to changes without rocking one's entire foundation. Nonetheless, exposure to a wider philosophy of health care is necessary at all levels if true change is to occur.

While the American public hotly debates the current issue of what format orthodox Western medicine will take, as was said before, this is the same product, albeit it with different packaging. It is already clear in data gathered from the British National Health Service that the fundamental assumptions of Western health care are flawed. In the early twentieth century Albert Beveridge formulated the British system based on the following assumption: that there exists in every population a strictly limited amount of morbidity which, if treated under conditions of equity, will eventually decline.[1] Thus it was calculated that the annual cost of the British National Health Service would fall as therapy reduced the rate of illness.[2]

Needless to say, this reduction in health-care dollars has not occurred in the British system nor anywhere else in Western industrialized medicine. And unfortunately, until the patient is reempowered with the ability for autonomous healing, we will never see that promised reduction in health-care expenditure. Nothing less than the complete radicalization of present medical education, similar to what I have suggested, will even begin to confront the problem at its most fundamental level.

Fortunately or unfortunately, for actively growing persons, be they health-care providers or not, education never stops. One of the greatest shocks one will encounter after graduation is the continuing evolution of one's practice. It never ceases to amaze me that month by month, year by year I have become a different practitioner; that virtually all of my surgical techniques and many of my medical interventions are radically different from what they were five years ago.

Change is the hallmark of evolution. And since we all seem to be involved in an evolutionary process both as individuals and as a planet, we must confront the concept of change bravely. My only hope is that in providing this information, I have made it easier for all of us to accept the necessary steps that must occur.

> "'A doctor is not merely a dispenser and synthesizer of scientific knowledge, nor is a patient an inert receptacle.' As Norman Cousins said, 'Ultimately it is the physician's respect for the human soul that determines the worth of his science.'"[3]

May this inspire you to provide and/or achieve perfect health, peace, and happiness.

God bless!

Appendix A

Just prior to publication of this book, I had a random sampling of friends — some patients, some physicians — review the manuscript. The lay people and paramedical personnel (certified technicians) uniformly agreed with the book's basic principles and were enthusiastic about the treatment possibilities it suggested. The reviewing physicians, on the other hand, appeared somewhat defensive and confused. The physicians specifically had a very hard time with the chapter on naturopathy.

In trying to decide why there was such a large disparity between the two reading audiences, I came to realize that patients are intuitively more in tune with the concept of natural healing. Most elderly patients I see in the office are convinced that they are overmedicated and treated in a piecemeal fashion with no concern for the big picture. Given the choice, as I have related elsewhere in the book, most patients delight at the thought of a more natural treatment, which will allow their bodies to heal themselves.

Most physicians, on the other hand, have erroneously come to believe that they heal by intervention. This is not hard to understand, as many of the medical situations they tackle are truly end-stage diseases, acute emergencies, or life-threatening illnesses. In these instances, intervention and control are necessary. However, so accustomed have physicians become to thinking in this manner that the entire relationship between doctor/controller/interventionist and the body's own natural protective healing mechanisms is lost.

All of the alternative medical systems reviewed here have in common that they set up a condition to allow nature to heal the body itself with a minimum of physician intervention. I believe that with a slight adjustment to our thinking we, as allopathic physicians, can learn to do the same thing. We can learn to withhold traditional interventions (taking control) except in cases of extreme medical emergencies or end-stage diseases alone. I again remind the physicians of the wisdom of Hippocrates: "Nature is the healer of disease. Nature itself finds means and ways. The task of the physician is to help nature in any way he can, not to try to do too much himself, but to make it possible for nature to effect her cure."[1]

Appendix B

The following is a list of resources for those who wish to obtain more information regarding a certain alternative medical system elucidated in this text. These resources will be listed alphabetically and not in the order of the chapters in which they appeared:

ACUPRESSURE:
Acupressure Institute
1533 Shattuck Avenue
Berkeley, CA 94709
(510) 845-1059

ACUPUNCTURE:
**American Academy of
Medical Acupuncture**
4820 Wilshire Boulevard,
Suite 500
Los Angeles, CA 90036
(213) 937-5514

**American Association of
Acupuncture and Oriental
Medicine**
4101 Lake Boone Trail
Raleigh, NC 27607
(919) 787-5181

**American Foundation of
Traditional Chinese Medicine**
1280 Columbus Avenue, Suite 302
San Francisco, CA 94133
(415) 776-0502

California Acupuncture Association
2180 Garnet Avenue, Suite 3G1
San Diego, CA 92109
(800) 477-4564

International Foundation of Oriental Medicine
4262 Kissena Boulevard
Flushing, NY 11355
(718) 321-8642

APPLIED KINESIOLOGY:
Biokinesiology Institute
5432 Highway 227
Trail, OR 97541
(503) 878-2080

International College of Applied Kinesiology, USA
P.O. Box 905
Lawrence, KS 66044
(913) 542-1801

AYURVEDA:
Maharishi Ayurvedic Association of America
P.O. Box 282
Fairfield, IA 52556
(515) 472-8477

CHIROPRACTIC:
National Association for Chiropractic Medicine
(713) 280-8262

Orthopractic Manipulation Society International
P.O. Box 145
Beaconsfield, Quebec, Canada
H9W 5T7

HERBALISM:
American Botanical Council
P.O. Box 201660
Austin, TX 78720
(512) 331-8868 or (800) 373-7105

American Herbalist Guild
P.O. Box 1863
Soquel, CA 95073-1863
(408) 438-1700

American Herb Association
P.O. Box 1673
Nevada City, CA 95959
(916) 265-9552

Herb Research Foundation
1007 Pearl Street, Suite 200
Boulder, CO 80302
(303) 449-2265

Herb Society of America
9019 Kirtland Chardon Road
Mentor, OH 44060
(216) 256-0514

HOMEOPATHY:
Homeopathic Association of Naturopathic Physicians
14653 Graves Road
Mulino, OR 97042
(503) 829-7326

Homeopathic Educational Services
2124 Kittridge Street
Berkeley, CA 94704
(510) 649-0294

International Foundation for Homeopathy
2366 Eastlake Avenue East, Suite 301
Seattle, WA 98102
(206) 324-8230

National Center for Homeopathy
801 North Fairfax Street, Suite 306
Alexandria, VA 22314
(703) 548-7790

MACROBIOTIC:
East/West Foundation
Macrobiotic Headquarters
P.O. Box 850
Brookline, MA 02146
(617) 738-0045

George Ohsawa
Macrobiotic Foundation
1511 Robinson Street
Oroville, CA 95965
(916) 533-7703

Kushi Institute of the Berkshires
P.O. Box 7
Becket, MA 01223
(413) 623-5741

MEDITATION:
TRANSCENDENTAL MEDITATION
CENTERS M.V.U.: FOR THE MOST
CURRENT LOCATION AND PHONE
NUMBERS CALL **1-800-843-8332**

4302 N. 44th Street
P.O. Box 80332
Phoenix, AZ 85060-0332
(312) 954-9292

944 W. 11th Avenue
Anchorage, AK 99501
(907) 258-6261

2716 Derby Street
Berkeley, CA 94705
(415) 548-1144

470 San Antonio Road
Palo Alto, CA 94306
(415) 857-0162

2168 Balboa Avenue, #2
San Diego, CA 92109
(619) 272-6500

1013 South 9th Street
Fargo, ND 58103
(701) 232-6162

19474 Center Ridge Road
Rocky River, OH 44116
(216) 333-6700

1391 S. Pennsylvania Street
Denver, CO 80210-2228
(303) 722-5076

19 Prospect Hill Road
Stony Creek, CT 06495
(203) 483-5180

1961 S. Columbia
Seaside, OR 97138
(503) 292-4034

234 South 22nd Street
Philadelphia, PA 19103
(215) 732-8464

P.O. Box 366715
San Juan, PR 00936-6715
(809) 722-8585

141 Waterman Street
Providence, RI 02906
(401) 751-1518

13789 Noel Road, Suite 116
Dallas, TX 75240
(214) 387-8686

1032 Eastwood Avenue
Salt Lake City, UT 84105
(801) 359-8686

4317 Linden Avenue N.
Seattle, WA 98103
(206) 547-7527

18682 East 17th Street
Santa Ana, CA 92705
(714) 832-0328

1018 Garden Street, #108
Santa Barbara, CA 93101
(805) 962-8916

2750 Spanish River Road
Boca Raton, FL 33432-8141
(407) 392-5418

P.O. Box 2550
1125 S.W. 2nd Avenue
Gainesville, FL 32601
(904) 338-1249

250 Sandspur Road
Maitland, FL 32751
(407) 539-2241

155 Stewart Drive N.E.
Atlanta, GA 30342
(404) 250-9560

2407 Parker Place
Honolulu, HI 96822
(808) 988-2266

636 South Michigan Ave.
Chicago, IL 60657
(312) 431-0110

3434 N. Washington Boulevard
Indianapolis, IN 46205
(317) 923-2873

33 Garden Street
Cambridge, MA 0218
(617) 876-4581

6301 Main Street
Kansas City, MO 64113
(816) 523-5777

600 Camden Avenue
Moorestown, NJ 08057-2242
(609) 231-0955

12 West 21st Street, 9th Floor
New York, NY 10011
(212) 645-0202

234 Culvert Road
Rochester, NY 14607
(716) 244-0434

In Canada
R.R. #2
Huntsville, ONT P0A 1K0
(705) 635-2234

1235 17th Avenue S.W. #308
Calgary, ALB T2T 0C2
(403) 229-0406

6076 East Boulevard
Vancouver, BC V6M 3V5
(604) 263-2655

1498 Younge Street, #203
Toronto, ONT M4T 1Z6
(416) 964-1725

220 Grand Allee, E #250
Quebec City, QUE G1R 2J1
(418) 529-8464

4205 St. Denis, #320
Montreal, QUE H2J 2K9
(514) 288-7704

NAPRAPATHY:

American Naprapathic Association
5913 W. Montrose Avenue
Chicago, IL 60641
(312) 685-6020

National College of Naprapathy
3330 N. Milwaukee Avenue
Chicago, IL 60641
(312) 282-5717

NATUROPATHY:

**American Association of
Naturopathic Physicians**
P.O. Box 20386
Seattle, WA 98102
(206) 323-7610

John Bastyr College
144 N.E. 54th Street
Seattle, WA 98105
(206) 523-9585

**National College of
Naturopathic Medicine**
11231 S.E. Market Street
Portland, OR 97216
(503) 255-4860

Footnotes

CHAPTER 1:

1. Eisenberg, D. M., R. C. Kessler, C. Foster, et al., "Unconventional Medicine in the United States. Prevalence, Costs, and Patterns of Use" *New England Journal of Medicine*, 1993, January 28; 328(4): pp. 246-252.

2. Maslow, Abraham, *Towards a Psychology of Being*, Princeton, N.J., Von Nostrand, 1968.

3. Griggs, Barbara, *Green Pharmacy: The History and Evolution of Western Medicine*, Rochester, Vt., Healing Arts Press, 1981, 1991, p. X in Foreword by Norman R. Farnsworth.

4. Ibid, p. 286, citing "Task Force on Preparation of Drugs: Final Report U.S. Department of Health, Education & Welfare," *Modern Medicine*, p. 35.

5. Illich, Ivan, *Medical Nemesis: The Expropriation of Health*, New York, Random House, Inc., 1976, p. 1.

6. Griggs, Barbara, Ibid, p. 289, citing Milton Silverman, *The Drugging of the Americas*, Berkeley, Calif., 1976.

7. Illich, Ibid, pp. 34-35.

8. Ibid, pp. 261-262.

9. Ibid, p. 39.

10. Piaget, Jean, *The Child's Conception of the World*, Translated by Joan & Andrew Tomlinson, Totowa, N.J., Littlefield, Adams & Co., 1969, p. 29.

11. Mendelsohn, Robert S., MD, *Confessions of a Medical Heretic*, New York, Warner Books Edition, 1980, pp. 13-14 & 17.

CHAPTER 2:

1. Illich, Ivan, *Medical Nemesis: The Expropriation of Health*, New York, Random House, Inc., 1976, p. 7.

2. Ibid, p. 9.

3. Ibid, p. 42.

4. Classen, D. C., et al., *JAMA*, 11/27/91, Vol. 266, No. 20.

5. Davis, Adelle, *Let's Eat Right to Keep Fit*, New York, Harcourt Brace, 1970.

6. Kastner, Mark, L.Ac., Dipl.Ac., & Hugh Burroughs, *Alternative Healing*, La Mesa, Calif., Halcyon Publishing, 1993, pp. 147-148.

7. Ibid, p. 14-15.

8. Ibid, p. 15.

9. Murray, Michael T., ND, *The Healing Power of Herbs*, Rocklin, Calif., Prima Publishing, 1992.

10. Murray, Michael, ND, & Joseph Pizzorno, ND, *Encyclopedia of Natural Medicine*, Rocklin, Calif., Prima Publishing, 1991.

CHAPTER 3:

1. Singh, S. J., *History and Philosophy of Naturopathy*, Lucknow, The Nature Cure Printarium, 1980, p. 40.

2. Ibid, p. 274.

3. Ibid, p. 532.

4. Ibid, p. 533.

5. Ibid, p. 548.

6. Ibid, p. 589.

7. Lerner, Michael, *Choices in Healing*, MIT Press, Cambridge, Mass, 1994.

CHAPTER 4:

1. Kennett, Frances, *Folk Medicine: Fact and Fiction*, New York, Crescent Books, 1976, p. 43.

2. Griggs, Barbara, *Green Pharmacy: The History and Evolution of Western Herbal Medicine*, Rochester, Vt., Healing Arts Press, 1981, 1991, p. 177.

3. Ibid, pp. 176-186.

4. Ibid, p. 238.

5. Ibid, p. 239.

6. Bayley, Calif. rol, *Homeopathy*, citing J. C. Calif. zin, et al.: 1987, "A study of the effect of decimal and centesimal dilution of arsenic on retention and mobilization of arsenic in the rat," *Human Toxicology* 6, pp. 315-320.

7. Ibid, citing C. Day: 1984, "Control of stillbirths in pigs using homeopathy," *Veterinary Record*, pp. 114 and 216.

8. Ibid, citing P. Fisher, et al., 1989, "Effect of homeopathic treatment on fibrositis (primary fibromyalgia)," *British Medical Journal*, pp. 229 and 365-366.

9. Ibid, citing D. T. Reilly, et al.: 1986, "Is homeopathy a placebo response: Controlled trial of potency, with pollen in hayfever as model," *Lancet 2*, pp. 881886.

10. Kleignen, J. and P. Knipschild, et al., "Clinical Trials of Homeopathy," *British Medical Journal*, 1991, Feb. 9, Vol. 302(6772), pp. 316-323.

11. Bayley, Carol, Ibid, citing Wiesenauer and Gaus, 1985, p. 143.

12. Ibid, citing A. Sacks: 1983, "Nuclear magnetic resonance spectroscopy of homeopathic remedies," *Journal of Holistic Medicine* 5, pp. 172-175.

13. James, G., "Homeopathy: An Energy Level of Therapy," *Professional Nurse*, Vol. 9, No. 1, 1993, pp. 54-57.

CHAPTER 5:

1. Griggs, Barbara, *Green Pharmacy: The History and Evolution of Western Herbal Medicine*, Rochester, Vt., Healing Arts Press, 1981, 1991, p. I in Foreword by Norman R. Farnsworth.

2. Ibid, p. 294.

3. Ibid, p. 295.

4. Kennett, Frances, *Folk Medicine: Fact and Fiction*, New York, Crescent Books, 1976, pp. 46-47.

5. David Kessler, FDA Commissioner, speaking on "Larry King Live," 1992.

6. Schulick, Paul, *Common Spice or Wonder Drug? Ginger: Health Care Rediscovers Its Roots,* Brattleboro, Vt. Herbal Free Press, 1993, p. 67, citing R. McCaleb, "Rational Regulation of Herbal Products Testimony Before the Subcommittee on Government Regulations," citing *Innovations in Medicine* No. 17, Pharmaceutical Manufacturers Association.

7. Ibid, p. 68, citing Annual Meeting: Federation of American Societies for Experimental Biology, New Orleans, La., March 31, 1993 (confirmed by two other high officials).

8. Illich, Ivan, *Medical Nemesis: The Expropriation of Health,* New York, Random House, Inc., 1976, p. 42.

CHAPTER 6:

1. Beideman, R. P., BA, DC, *Chiropractic History,* Vol. 3, No. 1, 1983, pp. 17-23.

2. Ibid.

3. American Medical Association, Opinions and Reports of the Judicial Council, December 31, 1960.

4. *Consumer Reports,* June 1994, Vol. 59, No. 6, N.Y., Consumers Union of U.S., Incorporated, p. 389.

5. Ibid.

6. Beck, Mark, *The Theory and Practice of Therapeutic Massage,* Albany, N.Y., Milady Publishing Company, 1988, pp. 3-12.

CHAPTER 7:

1. Kastner, Mark, L.Ac., Dipl.Ac., and Hugh Burroughs, *Alternative Healing,* La Mesa, Calif., Halcyon Publishing, 1993, p. 4.

2. Omura, Yoshiaki, ScD, MD, *Acupuncture Medicine: Its Historical and Clinical Background,* Tokyo, Japan Publications, Inc., 1982, p. 28.

3. Ibid, pp. 259-262.

4. Ibid, p. 260.

5. Ibid, p. 260.

6. Ibid, p. 261.

7. Kastner, Mark, Ibid, pp. 36.

8. Chopra, Deepak, MD, *Perfect Health: The Complete Mind/Body Guide,* New York, Harmony Books, 1991, p. 6.

9. Ibid, p. 3.

10. Ibid, p. 24.

11. Ibid, pp. 33-40.

12. Ibid, pp. 72-73.

13. Ibid, p. 171.

14. Orme Johnson, David W., Ph.D., & John T. Farrow, Ph.D., eds. *Scientific Research on the Transcendental Meditation Program*, Collect Papers, Volume I, West Germany, MERU Press, 1977.

15. Citing Bill Moyers's PBS Television Special "Healing and the Mind," 1993, copyright by Public Affairs Television, Inc., and David Grubin Productions, Inc.

CHAPTER 8:

1. Leviton, Richard, "What Does Illness Mean?" *Yoga Journal*, November/December 1991, Escondido, Calif., pp. 5051.

2. Capra, Fritjof, *Tao of Physics*, New York, Random House, 1983.

3. Benor, Daniel J., "Survey of Spiritual Healing Research," *Complimentary Medical Research* No. 4:1, September 1990, pp. 933.

4. Cited p. 18 of the Foreword, John White, *The Meeting of Science and Spirit: Guidelines* for a New Age, New York, Paragon House, 1990, p. 100.

5. Orme Johnson, David W., Ph.D., and John T. Farrow, Ph.D., eds., Scientific Research on the *Transcendental Meditation Program*, Collected Papers, Vol. I, West Germany, MERU Press, 1977.

6. Science of Creative Intelligence as taught by Maharishi Mahesh Yogi.

7. Plato, *The Republic* as translated by Paul Shorey, reprinted in *The Collected Dialogues of Plato*, Edith Hamilton and Huntington Carns, eds., Princeton University Press, 1973, pp. 50 & 64.

CHAPTER 9:

1. Mahesh Yogi, Maharishi, *The Science of Being and Art of Living*, London, International SRM Publications, 1963.

2. Eisenberg, D. M., R. C. Kessler, C. Foster, et al., "Unconventional Medicine in the United States. Prevalence, Costs, and Patterns of Use," *New England Journal of Medicine*, 1993, January 28; 328(4): pp. 246-252.

3. As a certified teacher of the Transcendental Meditation program since 1975, I can attest to the fact that no alteration of lifestyle nor conflict

with religious belief is necessary for the practice of this meditation. However, a small group of disgruntled students and teachers believe the opposite is true. They feel that both their lifestyles and religious beliefs have been challenged by this technique and published their dissatisfaction in a newsletter called *TM-EX*.

4. The basic Transcendental Meditation technique is taught for a practice of twenty minutes twice a day. Advanced courses featuring longer periods of meditation are offered to practitioners as an option, but are by no means necessary.

5. Orme Johnson, David W., Ph.D., and John T. Farrow, Ph.D., eds., *Scientific Research on the Transcendental Meditation Program*, Collected Papers, Vol. 1, West Germany: MERU Press, 1977.

6. Chopra, Deepak, MD, *Perfect Health: The Complete Mind/Body Guide*, New York, Harmony Books, 1991, and *Ageless Body, Timeless Mind: The Quantum Alternative to Growing Old*, New York, Harmony Books, 1993.

CHAPTER 10:

1. Shulick, Paul, *Common Spice or Wonder Drug? Ginger: Health Care Rediscovers Its Roots*, Brattleboro, Vt., Herbal Free Press, 1993, p. 64, citing 1990 GAO Report, Washington, D.C.

2. Ibid, p. 62, citing FDA Task Force Report, Washington, D.C., June 15, 1993.

3. Ibid, p. 68, citing 1990 GAO Report, Washington, D.C.

4. Griggs, Barbara, *Green Pharmacy: The History and Evolution of Western Medicine*, Rochester, Vt., Healing Arts Press, 1981, 1991, p. 112.

5. Ibid, p. 113.

6. Carter, J. A., *Racketeering in Medicine: The Suppression of Alternatives*, Hampton Roads, 1992, citing Dr. David Eddy, Director, Duke University Health Policy Research.

7. Cotts, Cynthia, *The Nation*, Aug. 3/Sept. 7, 1992, citing Eugene Robbins, MD, Professor Emeritus, Stanford University.

8. C. Everett Koop, MD, Former U.S. Surgeon General, cited in *New York Times*, Sept. 22, 1992.

9. Schulick, Paul, Ibid, p. 3, citing *Eating Well*, March-April 1993, p. 51.

10. Illich, Ivan, *Medical Nemesis: The Expropriation of Health*, New York, Random House, Inc., 1976, pp. 274-275.

CHAPTER 11:

1. Ibid, p. 221, citing Henry E. Sigerist, "From Bismarck to Beveridge: Developments and Trends in Social Security Legislation," *Bulletin of the History of Medicine* 13 (April 1943: 365-88).

2. Ibid, p. 221, citing Office of Health *Economics, Prospects in Health,* Publication No. 37 (London, 1971).

3. Dossey, Larry, MD, *Healing Words: The Power of Prayer and the Practice of Medicine,* New York, HarperCollins, 1993, p. 133, citing Paul Roud, "Making Miracles."

APPENDIX A:

1. Singh, S. J., *History and Philosophy of Naturopathy,* Lucknow, The Nature Cure Printarium, 1980, p. 40.

About the Author

Dr. Sarnat is an active physician in private practice throughout the Chicago metropolitan area. He has offices in Highland Park, Blue Island, and Palos Heights, Illinois. This is rather unique as his office clientele comes from blue-collar areas on Chicago's South Side and from the wealthiest communities on the North Shore. Dr. Sarnat specializes in ophthalmology, the medical and surgical care of the eye, with a special interest in pediatric ophthalmology.

He received his undergraduate education at Washington University in St. Louis, where he had a triple major in philosophy, psychology, and premedical sciences. He graduated magna cum laude in philosophy, his primary major, and he was elected to Phi Beta Kappa. Given his excellent academic achievements as an undergraduate, he was nominated by the university to be in contention for Rhodes and Oxford scholarships. However, Dr. Sarnat declined the offer in order to pursue medicine directly. He graduated from Rush Medical College in Chicago and completed his ophthalmic residency at Northwestern University. He is an active member in the American Medical Association as well as American Academy of Ophthalmology.

Dr. Sarnat has been politically active in the controversial area of the relationship between optometry and ophthalmology. He is one of the founders and active partners in the Midwest Eye Institute, which is a unique co-management center run jointly by both ophthalmologists and optometrists. It represents a futuristic model of cooperation between two health-care specialties that have traditionally been in competition.

— Dr. Sarnat is also actively involved with the research, development, and manufacture of various health-food commodities. He has an active interest in the development of food-bound vitamins, herbal medicines, natural skin-care products and the use of nontraditional medical-supplements.

Practicing what he preaches, Dr. Sarnat tries to lead a balanced life that includes daily meditation, a vegetarian diet, and regular exercise. He would cite his primary goals in life as the personal achievement of perfect health and the promotion of the highest possible level of health worldwide. He hopes this book will provide the social, political, and medical stimulus to realize this achievement more quickly.